SPIRITUAL HEALING

SPIRITUAL HEALING

Science, Meaning, and Discernment

EDITED BY
SARAH COAKLEY

WILLIAM B. EERDMANS PUBLISHING COMPANY
GRAND RAPIDS, MICHIGAN

Wm. B. Eerdmans Publishing Co.
4035 Park East Court SE, Grand Rapids, Michigan 49546
www.eerdmans.com

26 25 24 23 22 21 20   1 2 3 4 5 6 7

ISBN 978-0-8028-7093-3

Library of Congress Cataloging-in-Publication Data

Names: Coakley, Sarah, 1951– editor.
Title: Spiritual healing : science, meaning, and discernment / edited by Sarah
    Coakley.
Description: Grand Rapids, Michigan : William B. Eerdmans Publishing Com-
    pany, 2020. | Includes bibliographical references and index. | Summary:
    "An interdisciplinary assessment of the phenomenon of spiritual healing" —
    Provided by publisher.
Identifiers: LCCN 2020016399 | ISBN 9780802870933 (paperback)
Subjects: LCSH: Spiritual healing. | Healing — Religious aspects.
Classification: LCC BL65.M4 S6735 2020 | DDC 203/.1 — dc23
LC record available at https://lccn.loc.gov/2020016399

Unless otherwise noted, quotations from Scripture are taken from the New
Revised Standard Version of the Bible.

*This book is dedicated, with gratitude and admiration,
to Mary Ann Meyers, gracious and patient enabler
of the science and religion debates.*

Contents

PART THREE
PHILOSOPHICAL INSIGHTS

PART FOUR
ANTHROPOLOGICAL AND PASTORAL PERSPECTIVES

Introduction

Spiritual Healing, Science, and Meaning

Sarah Coakley

The Scope of This Book

This is a book about spiritual healing, its significance in today's medical and cultural worlds, its understanding in scientific terms, and its meaning and explanation in theological categories. It will be of equal interest to the general reading public and to specialists whose disciplines are utilized in it. After all, no one in this life escapes the threat of illness, distress, disease, and ultimately death; the elusive prospect of healing, from whatever ails one, therefore has a certain timeless and universal allure.

The scope of this book is thus both ambitious, in interdisciplinary terms, and yet also intentionally focused, in what it sets out to explore and clarify. Its main interest is in how *meaning-ascription* and *interpretation* of healing events provide a crucial underlying fulcrum for the efficacy of healing. But this is not, as we shall see, the same thing as reducing healing to wish-fulfillment, let alone to self-delusion; even at the level of brain-event, it can now be shown neuroscientifically that interpretation plays a key role in the experience of pain and illness, and thus also in the alleviation or transformation of these states.[1] Sometimes phenomena such as these are clustered under the rather flexible and

1. See especially Howard L. Fields's contribution in this book (chapter 4), and also his important earlier companion essay, "Setting the Stage for Pain: Allegorical Tales from Neuroscience," in *Pain and Its Transformations: The Interface of Biology and Culture*, ed. Sarah Coakley and Kay Kaufman Shelemay (Cambridge, MA: Harvard University Press, 2007), 36–61.

contested category of placebo;[2] but as the essays in this book will demonstrate, this is by no means always the case, nor need it be. *All* experiences of disease and healing come with meanings attached; the interesting thing is what shifts those meanings and with what effect.

A distinct, but obviously related, issue is under what conditions it is rational to ascribe a healing to some metaphysical force *beyond* the realm open to investigation by empirical science and medicine.[3] Here perforce we enter the speculative fields of philosophy, philosophy of science, and theology. But as this volume will also demonstrate, there is a great variety of philosophical and theological models available for thinking about resolutions of illness or disease that appear not to accord with medical expectation, and not all of them are explicitly *theistic*. When they are theistic, much then depends — in seeking to provide a fuller theological account of them — on exactly how the relation between God and the world is construed.[4] In the course of the essays that unfold here, a number of different ways of thinking about natural and supernatural healings will be discussed, rendering questionable the assumption made by many contemporary scientists that the only theological alternative to a medically explicable healing event is a purported act of God that explicitly defies and flouts modern scientific presumptions altogether.[5] Indeed, not only is this

2. See Anne Harrington's work in this volume (chapter 6), and more fully in Anne Harrington, ed., *The Placebo Effect: An Interdisciplinary Exploration* (Cambridge, MA: Harvard University Press, 1997). As we shall note later in this introduction, and as Harrington herself discusses, the term *placebo* can cover a confusingly wide variety of phenomena, from its technical meaning as an inert pill to the confidence instilled in a patient by an attentive and sympathetic medical practitioner.

3. This issue is discussed variously in this book by Howard L. Fields (chapter 4), who mentions the presumption in the scientific world that a nonempirical cause would be considered only if all other possibilities of explanation had been exhausted; by Anne Harrington (chapter 6), who contests this view and describes it as manifesting an unfortunate "eliminative logic"; and by Philip Clayton (chapter 7), who provides a sustained discussion of how to adjudicate between the various "metaphysical" claims that are raised by the phenomenon of spiritual healing.

4. This issue is discussed illuminatingly by Philip Clayton (chapter 7). I engage his views and offer a further alternative in the section below entitled "The Texture of Theological Accounts of Spiritual Healing."

5. This is sometimes called the "combat" model of the relation of science and theology, and is critiqued by a number of contributors in this book, including Anne Harrington in her discussion of medical "prayer experiments" (chapter 6). It is, however, an irony that the official Roman Catholic view on miracles explicitly leans on this same modernistic presumption that an event can be termed miraculous only if all other medical and scientific explanations have failed: see the discussion by Emma Anderson (chapter 2), pp. 54–56.

disjunctive alternative an unnecessary one scientifically; it is also one that may not represent the most subtle theological option on offer either. I shall return to a more substantial discussion of this theological issue in a later section of this introduction; but suffice it here to note in anticipation that the various choices to be made in explaining spiritual healing lead not only, and inexorably, into metaphysical reflection of various sorts but also into important areas of spiritual and moral discernment: assessing the spiritual significance and ethical import of healings is not an optional addendum to the issues discussed here but often a key factor in an evaluation of their wider cultural or religious importance.

What *Is* Spiritual Healing? A Semantic Clarification

We cannot proceed further in this introduction to the book's aims and goals, however, without a somewhat chastening semantic clarification of what *spiritual healing* connotes and how the authors in this volume have been required to specify their task in illuminating it. Perhaps it will be clear from what I have written already that at least one crucial ambiguity in the use of the term *spiritual healing* is unavoidable but needs careful comment nonetheless.

The term *spiritual healing*, that is, may simply refer, first, to any healing that is not strictly physical, that is, which relates to the psychic, or non-somatic, or spiritual elements of the self. On this definition, it is the *locus* of the healing that is being described as spiritual. Of course it need not follow on this definition that the body is not also affected in any such healing (indeed the apparently intrinsic unity of the psychosomatic self makes it likely that there will also be at least some somatic effect);[6] but the point here is that the primary focus of interest lies in the psychic or spiritual event of healing in the self. A number of the essayists in this book focus almost entirely on this first rendition of spiritual healing.[7] They do so because they do not themselves wish to speculate

6. Philosophy of mind issues therefore cannot be avoided in this discussion either, and indeed in medical research more generally: see Philip Clayton (chapter 7), who also reflects in detail on the mind/body distinction and provides a range of different possible contemporary positions that may be taken on the philosophy of mind issue.

7. These include the historians Emma Anderson and Heather D. Curtis (chapters 2 and 3), the neuroscientist Howard L. Fields (chapter 4), the neuroscientist/psychologist Malcolm Jeeves (chapter 5), the historian of science Anne Harrington (chapter 6), and the anthropologist Thomas Csordas (chapter 9). Philip Clayton's work (chapter 7) is in contrast particularly concerned with how *legitimately* to move from "spiritual dimensions of healing" to claims for "spiritual [sc. divine] healing" per se.

theologically or perhaps do not regard themselves as competent to do so; but they nonetheless think that there are plenty of illuminating things to say about spiritual healings, *qua* human events. There are usually also correlative things to say about how these human events have *social* location and meaning as well; in these contexts, one may then speak of the spiritual dimensions of healing.

A second rendition of spiritual healing, in contrast, refers to a healing that is effected directly by God (or by other purported spiritual forces), or by God assisted by human others, secondarily and cooperatively. On this definition, it is the *source* of the healing event that is being described as spiritual (that is, God or the divine). It will be clear immediately that these two meanings of spiritual healing are not mutually exclusive (although one refers to the *locus*, and the other to the *source*, as spiritual): where the latter is at stake, the former will almost always be involved as well. But it is important again to note that the former may be discussed on its own — and with considerable intellectual profit — without any specific presumptions being made about the latter. The interest then comes in bringing these discussions together, as is attempted in this book; but the initial distinction remains vital.

One of the reasons why it is hard to keep these different definitions strictly distinct, however, is that the related noun *spirituality* — now so popular and so widely and ambiguously used — drops a pall of confusion, even mystification, on the whole matter and thus makes it difficult *ab initio* to maintain clarity about what might be involved in a spiritual healing. A word of caution about this term, too, is therefore necessary at this point, even though it is not much utilized in this book.[8]

The noun *spirituality* is a relatively modern one, in contrast to the adjective *spiritual* (*pneumatikos* in Greek), which is used very commonly in the New Testament and earliest Christianity, and especially by Paul, to refer to the effects of the Holy Spirit on all Christians in virtue of their baptism.[9] Once the word started to be used regularly as a noun (much later, roughly from the Catholic Counter-Reformation period on),[10] it came to garner the specific technical

---

8. Indeed, almost entirely eschewed, under editorial caution!

9. See, for example, 1 Cor. 2:13–15; 3:1; and Paul's contentful teaching on the "law of the Spirit" (in which all Christians are *pneumatikoi* in virtue of their baptism), in Rom. 8:2–17.

10. A useful note on the history and meanings of the term *spirituality* appears in the preface of Cheslyn Jones, Geoffrey Wainwright, Edward Yarnold, SJ, eds., *The Study of Spirituality* (Oxford: Oxford University Press, 1986), xxii–xxvi. Simon Tugwell, *Ways of Imperfection: Exploration of Christian Spirituality* (Springfield, IL: Templegate Books, 1985), tells the history of Christian spirituality in a way precisely resistant to the commodification and elitism associated with the word *spirituality* becoming a noun from the Counter-Reformation period onward.

associations of ascetical theology, that is, that branch of theology that treats not of doctrine per se but of the theory and practice of prayer, meditation, contemplation, and accompanying practices of fasting, penitence, self-denial, and so on. In the contemporary period in the West, however, and particularly in popular parlance, the term *spirituality* has now come to accrue a bewildering array of meanings stretched well beyond this earlier ascetical and intra-Christian connotation. Indeed, an attraction to spirituality is often now understood to connote a primary interest in something only to be found in satisfactory form *outside* the churches: in types of spiritual practice, potentially elevated internal states, or other forms of psychic transformation sought specifically *out of relation to institutionalized religion* (as in the commonly cited tag, "I prefer spirituality, not religion").[11] For adherents to such a position, one of its attractions may be a release beyond any one particular religious tradition, or an eclectic use of several — perhaps with the hope that this will enable a transformative self-cultivation, an escape not only from religious authoritarianism but also from the corrosive effects of daily stress. Under these conditions, however, it may be particularly hard to clarify what, if any, specific metaphysical assertions are being made about the realm of spirituality, so-called — hence the potential blurring of the important distinction on the different meanings of spiritual healing, just explicated. Moreover, as one contributor to this volume opines in particular, there may also be a concomitant danger of what he calls "spookiness," that is, the appeal to a vague sense of transcendence that is not only devoid of any clear point of *metaphysical* reference but also comes without any obvious means of *moral* discernment of different states associated with the spiritual.[12] These points may seem, to some readers, unnecessarily harsh comments on the movements of spirituality now so popular, pervasive, and indeed influential in the contemporary West; but for the meantime, without prejudging the cultural significance of such new trends in general, it is simply to be noted that our task in this volume is to be as clear as possible about the reference and meaning of spiritual healing and to adjudicate with some exactitude the scientific, medical, metaphysical, and moral claims implied. The book will thus be read with as

11. On this phenomenon, see especially Paul Heelas and Linda Woodhead, with Benjamin Seel, Bronislaw Szerszynski, and Karin Tusting, *The Spiritual Revolution: Why Religion Is Giving Way to Spirituality* (Oxford: Blackwell, 2005); and Paul Heelas, ed., *Spirituality in the Modern World: Within Religious Tradition and Beyond* (London: Routledge, 2011). An instructive comparison of these studies with one in a North American (and historic New England) guise may be found in Courtney Bender, *The New Metaphysicals: Spirituality and the American Imagination* (Chicago: University of Chicago Press, 2010).

12. See Stephen R. L. Clark's discussion (chapter 8), pp. 154–60.

much profit by those engaged in forms of New Age spiritual practices as by those interested in more classical forms of religion.[13]

A final point of semantic clarification that needs to be made at the opening of this book relates to our other key term, *healing*. For this, too, is a multivalent notion; and perhaps the first and most important point of clarification here is that a healing may not necessarily connote a physical cure (although, of course, it can). But even a dying person can be healed in a significant sense relating to his or her psychic life, past experiences, or relationships with others, and this in turn may manifest itself in certain physical, albeit short-term, ameliorations of symptoms. Moreover, and cutting across this first distinction, healing may in some cases occur almost instantaneously and suddenly, or, rather differently, as part of a *process* of gradual transformation. And, finally, the *locus* of the ailment (and accompanying healing) may once again be varied: a specific bodily affliction, a mental illness, the effects of past abuse, a problem of unrepented sin, or a transindividual state of disorder (whether social, political, or institutional). One of the deeper complexities of healing, of course, is that these problems are often confusingly — and indeed unconsciously — intertwined. As we shall see, this gives extra significance to the problem of reordered *meaning* and *narrative* in the phenomenon of healing.

Cultural Contradictions and Spiritual Healing

Our discussion of the *semantic* complexity of the meaning of spiritual healing relates no less to its multifarious *cultural* significances in the postmodern West. Indeed, this study has been conducted at a time of marked "cultural contradiction" over matters of medicine and religion;[14] and this strange cultural phe-

---

13. A comparison with Fraser Watts, ed., *Spiritual Healing: Scientific and Religious Perspectives* (Cambridge: Cambridge University Press, 2011), 1–16, may be useful here in charting how different definitions of spiritual healing may variously be generated in parallel literature. Watts's first definition is "1. Healing in which spiritual practices play a role," and deliberately includes *any* such "practices" (not limiting them to Christianity). His other two definitions are roughly equivalent to the two I have rehearsed here, that is, "2. Healing in which spiritual aspects of the human are presumed to be involved"; and "3. Healing that is explained in terms of what are presumed to be spiritual processes" (p. 1). In effect, I have, in my own semantic analysis, included Watts's first definition within his second one; but like Watts, I see no reason why spiritual healing in this human sense should be restricted to those within classical religious traditions.

14. This is an illuminating term coined by the American sociologist Daniel Bell; see his renowned volume, *The Cultural Contradictions of Capitalism* (New York: Basic, 1976).

nomenon also seems to demand our critical attention at the outset of this book. As so often, a *frisson* of excitement and interest turns out to arise from deeply ambiguous roots.

On the one hand, one might say that Western biomedicine has never been more intellectually powerful, more confident in its technical advances, or more implicated in global patterns of economic privilege. On the other hand, perhaps never since the Enlightenment has there been such a huge — indeed, almost unchartable — explosion of alternative or complementary therapies, health regimes, spiritual practices, healing arts, fascination with the occult, and rampant religious eclecticism. It is as if the stern rigor and technicality of biomedical practice (its very touchstone of success) is nonetheless failing the human spirit at some basic points of need: for narrative meaning, for attention, for care, for the lure of the transcendent (however construed), and for the healing of soul as well as cure of body. Although in the United States the poor and marginalized, perforce, have little access (through underinsurance, or lack of it altogether) to the benefits of advanced biomedical technique, we should not make the mistake of presuming that alternative therapies are necessarily cheap. They too are subject to the notable postmodern phenomenon of the commodification of desire; and, perhaps more worryingly, they can also be inviting of undiscerning and gullible multiple-usage. Quackery — the medical skeptics say — has been rebaptized as complementary medicine; but this is an obvious oversimplification of a complex situation, in which dangerous and ignorant cranks may well be practicing alongside the most superb and highly trained experts in (say) historic Chinese acupuncture, whose efficacy and theoretic significance is not generally in doubt.[15] It is estimated that, overall, North Americans already spend at least a third as much money on alternative therapies as they do on their biomedical megalith; yet the latter has never before served so few, so expensively — albeit so masterfully.[16]

15. The work of David M. Eisenberg at Harvard Medical School has been particularly important in instigating research on the efficacy of Chinese medicine (including acupuncture) according to exacting biomedical standards; see Craig Lambert's article on Eisenberg's work, "The New Ancient Trend in Medicine: Scientific Scrutiny of 'Alternative' Therapies," *Harvard Magazine* (March–April 2002): 46–49, 99–101; and Eisenberg's publications, listed in the U. S. National Library of Medicine, https://www.ncbi .nlm.nih.gov/sites/myncbi/16y5oyfrfTWAm/bibliography/52315417/public/?sort=date &direction=descending.

16. Recent web-based information on the phenomenon of spending on alternative health therapies appears in Katherine Derla, "Americans Spend Billions on Alternative Medicine but Treatments Not Covered by Health Insurance," *Tech Times*, June 23, 2016, https://www.tech times.com/articles/166574/20160623/americans-spend-billions-on-alternative-medicine

To revert then to our earlier discussion of spirituality and its ambiguities, the situation of cultural contradiction we are now describing has parallel paradoxical dimensions: technical mastery versus eclectic gullibility; rich patients versus poor; secularism versus multiple New Age spiritualities; reductive physicalism versus resurgent dogmatic beliefs in the soul and the transcendent (from a variety of religious traditions): these disjuncts sit astride each other in postmodern North American society in endless varieties of conjunction, often coexisting confusingly in just one patient, family, or hospital. And well-established religious practitioners, too, are equally affected by these paradoxes, as becomes particularly clear in conditions of crisis in hospital.[17]

In *this* Western cultural context, then — not just in any context, I suggest — the notion of spiritual healing takes on new and peculiar allure. For somehow it promises what even the rich cannot buy and what even the biomedical megalith cannot explain: that pearl of great price — the healthy, whole, and perfected self. Yet even to summon that notion is immediately to highlight perhaps the greatest contemporary cultural contradiction of all, and not one that merely affects the realm of medicine and religion. For has not postmodern philosophy seen off the self, and has not neuroscience definitively reasserted the superior explanatory power of reductive physicalism?[18] Has not the body (that great obsession of the late twentieth century) finally replaced the elusive soul, and has not the notable American denial of death triumphed over individual eschatological hope?[19] Odd, then, that the language of soul/body should die so hard

---

-but-treatments-not-covered-by-health-insurance.htm. She points out that even those who are not insured medically are happy to spend significant funds on alternative medicines. In contrast, the money spent on standard clinical medical treatments in the United States is concentrated in a very small percentage of the population. See Bradley Sawyer and Gary Claxton (for the Kaiser Family Foundation), "How Do Health Expenditures Vary Across the Population?," Health System Tracker, January 16, 2019, https://www.healthsystemtracker .org/chart-collection/health-expenditures-vary-across-population/. I am grateful to Edith Coakley Stowe for professional assistance in charting this information, which does of course change from year to year.

17. My own experience as a hospital chaplain trainee in a Massachusetts Roman Catholic hospital (2000–2001) might be cited here by way of vignette. Chaplain interns such as myself (as opposed to Roman Catholic priests or nuns) were issued badges labeling us suppliers of "Spiritual Services," a nomenclature that in turn gave rise to an astonishing range of surprising conversations with those otherwise presumed to be traditional Roman Catholics. For a fascinating social-science account of how religious belief (and sometimes loss or lack of belief) plays out unexpectedly in hospital conditions of crisis, see Wendy Cadge, *Paging God: Religion in the Halls of Medicine* (Chicago: University of Chicago Press, 2012).

18. See Clayton's discussion of this issue (chapter 7), pp. 134–36.

19. See Jeffrey P. Bishop's searing analysis of the paradoxes of clinical medicine's attempt

culturally in the West, and that the notable striving for wholeness (a term of unexplained, but seemingly mantric, power) should almost always be linked to the rhetoric of a mind/body dualism. As I have written elsewhere, it is as if the disappearing smile of a Cartesian Cheshire cat still hovers over our Western obsessions with longevity, fitness, sexual performance, slimness — and healing. Can we still hope, perhaps, to orchestrate these bodily events from this other, remaining, site of control?[20] Yet the individualism of this Cartesian tradition is also in crisis just as it refuses to die: Why else should manifold corporate healing rituals spring up (many influenced by the Christian charismatic movement) to reassert the power of the divine, the communal and the transindividual, just at the same time as the verb *to heal*, strangely, has become an individualistic, intransitive one in popular psychobabble? "You must heal" has become a psychic demand, even for the lonely isolate. But that demand, too, comes with an implied moral narrative curiously hidden within it — in this case, a call to action, control, and self-improvement.

When Religion Enters the Medical Field of Healing: Some Caveats and Challenges

In this confused cultural context, it is barely surprising that religious narratives can often wend their way, almost by default, into the arena of spiritual healing, and in equally various and contestable ways. Some theoretical smoke also needs to be cleared here, then, and some means of discernment achieved, before we attack the more substantial doctrinal issue of explicitly *theological* explanatory models for healing events.

And here I must declare my own editorial hand. Despite — and one might say in the face of — the confusing cultural contradictions I have now outlined,

---

to reduce the body to inert flesh: *The Anticipatory Corpse: Medicine, Power, and the Care of the Dying* (Notre Dame: University of Notre Dame Press, 2011).

20. I discussed these cultural issues at some length in the introduction to my earlier volume, Sarah Coakley, ed., *Religion and the Body* (Cambridge: Cambridge University Press, 1997), 1–12, esp. 7. It is ironic that the objectification of the body, and the desire to control it from some other site, is as deeply engrained in lay Western consciousness as it is in the medical profession, where the *doctor's* attempt at mechanistic control of the body is both a core feature of the profession, and yet one often found distressing to the patient when it is not accompanied by empathy. For a sensitive discussion of this problem by an Anglican priest experienced in spiritual-healing practices, see Stephen Parsons, *Searching for Healing: Making Sense of the Many Paths to Wholeness* (Oxford: Lion, 1995), ch. 1.

and the profound difficulties of definition already faced, it seems to me that we currently confront an extraordinary transformation of consciousness in Western biomedical practice and research, which leaves ample room for new considerations of the significant place of religious narrative in relation to science (and specifically to medical science), where our disputed topic of spiritual healing is concerned.[21] But the huge danger at this point is to lurch too quickly to the gullible or superstitious end of the cultural spectrum, thus reinviting the scorn of the medical and philosophical guilds; whereas precisely what is needed is the most careful, sophisticated, and intellectually acute analysis — scientifically, philosophically, *and religiously*. It is this, I suggest, that must precede any otherwise hasty recourse to normative theological claims.

A number of particular arenas of healing that have attracted recent public discussion are revealing here, and — as we shall see — they are connected in their theoretic challenges. What conjoins these examples is some sort of attempt to introduce religious meaning systems into the biomedical realm of explanatory endeavor. What disjoins them is the extent to which the biomedical world has yet developed the theoretic religious insights to adjudicate what is at stake in terms of the implied truth claims and their veridicality; and here the contribution of medical anthropology (with its capacity to describe and assess the thick description of a healing event in context) may provide a particularly important exploratory bridge between the realm of medicine itself and any fully developed *theological* account of what may be happening.

The first task, then, would seem to be establishing that biomedicine itself has now arrived at a point where questions of spiritual healing (initially in the human spiritual sense, sketched above) are at least being broached. Several contributors to this volume are particularly well qualified to comment on different dimensions of these questions. Let us here draw attention to them in anticipation.

First, as already intimated above, recent developments in the neuroscientific investigation of pain suggest a new possible interface between top-down religious meaning systems and bottom-up neuroscientific explanations.[22] Once it

---

21. Recent publications that witness to this trend include Joan D. Koss-Chioino and Philip Hefner, eds., *Spiritual Transformation and Healing: Anthropological, Theological, Neuroscientific, and Clinical Perspectives* (Lanham, MD: AltaMira, 2006); the already mentioned Watts, *Spiritual Healing*; Harold G. Koenig, *Spirituality and Health Research: Methods, Measurements, Statistics, and Resources* (Philadelphia: Templeton, 2011); and Christopher Cook, ed., *Spirituality, Theology and Mental Health: Interdisciplinary Perspectives* (London: SCM, 2013).

22. Explanation and discussion of this crucial neuroscientific phenomenon, and its meaning, appears in this volume in the chapters by Howard L. Fields (chapter 4) and Malcolm

is acknowledged that the neural pathways conveying messages of local physical trauma to the brain in a pain experience never operate in isolation from *different* neural pathways that interpret that pain (and indeed that the latter pathways can be artificially provoked to induce an intense experience of so-called non-existent physical pain),[23] then we see how hermeneutics is becoming a new, key arena of mediation between neuroscience and the interpretative arts: philosophy, literature, and religion, among others. In other words, interpretation of pain can no longer be seen as an arbitrary *additum* (this is a misplaced, neo-Kantian disjunction), but rather something intrinsic both to our physiological experiences and to our scientific explanations — a bridge between physicalist explanation and lived experience.[24] More than one of our contributors note that this discovery might have spiraling effects for the broader area of mental health, in which religious meanings tend to have been dismissed as pathological by secular psychiatry's approach to psychosis.[25] The challenge, however, is not to announce on this basis, prematurely, the resistant *necessity* of the full-blown theological trope as a means of explanation; but rather, and more cautiously, it is to investigate the rich range of hermeneutical responses that an experience of pain or illness, whether physical or psychic, may produce, and how modifications to that pain may therefore potentially be effected without the use of explicitly medical interventions.[26]

Closely related to this finding is the huge, and mysterious, field of placebo research, also already mentioned at the outset of this introduction. A blanket

---

Jeeves (chapter 5). As Philip Clayton (chapter 7, pp. 146–47) sagely comments later, however, the nomenclature of "top-down" and "bottom-up" in scientific discussion has more than one application and important elements of philosophical ambiguity; for clarification, see the special journal issue, George F. R. Ellis, Dennis Noble, and Timothy O'Connor, eds., "Top-Down Causation," *Interface Focus* (February 2012); and in more detail, George F. R. Ellis, *How Can Physics Underlie the Mind? Top-Down Causation in the Human Context* (Berlin: Springer, 2016).

23. This is, of course, a misnomer, given the understanding we now have of the intricate mechanisms of the experience of pain: all felt pain *is* pain. See Coakley and Shelemay, *Pain and Its Transformations*, esp. 242–44.

24. This begins to explain how certain forms of physical illness particularly subject to intensification by anxiety (for example, heart disease, chronic problems with the immune system) may also be remarkably improved in some circumstances by the alleviation of fear, loneliness, and distress; see Watts, *Spiritual Healing*, esp. 132–33, on the developing field of "psychoneuroimmunology (PNI)."

25. See especially John Swinton's discussion (chapter 10) and his earlier book, *Spirituality and Mental Health Care: Rediscovering a 'Forgotten' Dimension* (London: Jessica Kingsley, 2001).

26. This issue is discussed in depth in Coakley and Shelemay, *Pain and Its Transformations*, pts. 2, 3, and 4.

term that currently may be used to cover inert doses in medical trials (its technical meaning), at one end of the spectrum, and spiritual healings (in either of the
senses outlined above), at the other, its fascinations clearly lie in investigating
the areas of trust, meaning, expectation, and hope in clinical well-being, and
the extraordinary power of positive or sympathetic interpretation for the experience of illness (including that of belief in religious meaning systems). Placebo
research therefore clearly admits the possibility of medically transformative
religious commitments;[27] but it also includes under its encompassing skirts the
importance for the sufferer of the kind of *attention* and *empathy* given to him or
her by the medical practitioner. And this too may involve an authentic willingness (or otherwise) of the practitioner to entertain the clinical importance of
religious narratives of explanation — or at least of trusting submission to divine
mystery — *for the patient*. Indeed, it has been hypothesized of late that the extraordinary success and cultural attraction of so-called complementary and alternative medicines may reside at least partly in the amount of time and sympathetic attention that the practitioner provides for the patient in these contexts,
in contrast to what tends to be the case in standard biomedical practice.[28]

Further, in cases such as yoga or acupuncture treatment where the original
context of the practice (India or China) was specifically religious and philosophical in its theory and assumptions, there is yet another reason why treatment may
be infused with religious paradigms and meanings. The subtle body, after all, is
one that Western biomedicine does not even entertain; but that does not mean
that it does not *exist*. Again, textured, discerning accounts both of medical theory and of patient experience are what are at stake in the further investigation
of the efficacy of classic Eastern alternative therapies.[29]

27. There may, of course, also be a *nocebo* dimension for religious people who fear death
and judgment, just as there can also be a beneficial religious *placebo* effect; see Anne Harrington's chapter 6.

28. Parsons, *Searching for Healing*, 17–21, draws attention to the dangers of doctors' abuse
of power in clinical practice and to the importance of the patient feeling some sense of personal
control during treatment, something often more catered for in alternative therapies (pp. 67–79).

29. For an important survey of current medical pluralism in the United States, see Ted J.
Kaptchuk and David M. Eisenberg, "Varieties of Healing. 1: Medical Pluralism in the United
States" and "Varieties of Healing. 2: A Taxonomy of Unconventional Healing Practices,"
Academia and Clinic: Complementary and Alternative Medicine Series, Annals of Internal Medicine
135 (2001): 189–95, 196–204. More recently, Jo Marchant, *Cure: A Journey into the Science of
Mind over Body* (New York: Broadway, 2016), presents a reliable, high-journalistic account
of the many ways in which holistic approaches to medicine are gaining scientific ground. In
relation to acupuncture specifically, a thick description of the Confucian theory of the self
and the meridians in the body, on which the practice of acupuncture is based, appears in Tu

So it does seem that at various levels of important current medical investigation of the experience of illness, religious narratives have a legitimate place and demand theoretic attention. In short, there is manifestly room for sophisticated discussion of religious meaning systems in *certain* kinds of medical research, as outlined here. But, second, and in contrast, there are at the same time profound theoretic dangers in developing these areas of research in ways that are tainted by (occluded) reductive scientistic presumptions, on the one hand, or by forms of theological naivete, on the other. Let me explain further.

This other side to the contested arena of medical healing and its relation to religion often reveals well-meaning attempts to demonstrate the importance of their relation while failing to realize the theoretic *complexity* of their interface. Indeed, still perhaps implicitly in thrall to the simplistic combat view of medical science and religion, medical practitioners may set up research agendas riddled with questionable assumptions, both scientific and theological. Two controversial and much-discussed examples may perhaps suffice to substantiate this thesis; what both demonstrate, as we shall see, is that a failure to attend to the thick description of the *experience* of sickness and healing from the perspective of the patient skews the protocol of such experiments from the outset. And this problem is only exacerbated if it is accompanied by a crude assumption about the possibility of *demarcating* a demonstrable act of God by merely statistical investigations of a complex medical scenario. Conversely, there are different sorts of problems if classic religious practices (which come front-loaded in their original contexts with deep — and often demanding — narratives of life, death, and transformative suffering) are reduced to a generic, secularized medical format designed for the mere alleviation of physical anxiety and discomfort. These two sets of problems may thus be seen as ironic mutual inversions: the first misleadingly *elevates* the possibility of theological meaning in a medical context, and the second *dilutes* it. But in neither case is the religious and theological complexity of the material at stake properly understood, nor is the wide diversity of patient experience — religious or otherwise — sufficiently reflected upon.[30]

In this volume, the first problem outlined here is discussed at some length by Anne Harrington (a historian and philosopher of science) in her incisive critique of a number of medical investigations on the force of intercessory prayer. As a

---

Weiming, "Pain and Humanity in the Confucian Learning of the Heart-and-Mind," in *Pain and Its Transformations*, ed. Coakley and Shelemay, 221–41.

30. This point is also made by Anne Harrington (chapter 6); and, in this book, the contribution by Thomas Csordas (chapter 9) most richly demonstrates the importance of sensitive *anthropological* study for exploring the richness and variety of religious responses to the crises of illness and healing.

theologian, however, I find it worth supplementing Harrington's account in advance by reference to an illuminating survey article on investigations of this sort, which already appeared in *The American Psychologist* in 2003.[31] What is troubling to the theologian, first, about the studies surveyed in this article is that religion is often assumed here (seemingly on principles derived from the work of William James) to be primarily about the affective, the internal, the noninstitutional, or nondogmatic; and hence some strain is evidenced when investigators admit that their subjects are often already fully embedded in religious institutions and their accompanying doctrinal commitments.[32] Spirituality, connectedly, appears to be an even more wafting category for the investigators, sometimes perceived quite naively as a sort of *private* religious high.[33] While some of these assumptions seemingly hold, also, for the psychologists conducting the relevant research, it is far from clear that the same applies to those being investigated, many of them being highly institutionalized Christian churchgoers with very firm doctrinal beliefs. So the protocols for the investigations appear to be distorted from the outset by the investigators' own presumptions. Again, the scientific assumption of most of the tests seems to be that *belief*, as such, has negligible intellectual — let alone neurological or psychological — significance; whereas blind testings of intercessory prayer, in contrast, can fall back on an almost magical understanding of transindividual efficacy, with absolutely no *theological* account given of the workings of intercession or cooperative grace, of the variables of personal openness of intercessors to divine action, of their own spiritual integrity, belief, and practices, and so on. Further, and finally, the extraordinarily crass assumption of many of the reported trials surveyed by Miller and Thorsen is that "living longer" is the prime sign of in-

31. William R. Miller and Carl E. Thorsen, "Spirituality, Religion, and Health: An Emerging Research Field," *American Psychologist* 58 (2003): 24–35. Note that I am not here directly criticizing the authors of this article as such (though it seems they share some of the presumptions they report, given that they offer no critical, alternative perspective). The article is mainly devoted to the laudable task of commending religion and spirituality as proper objects of scientific study, *contra* the objections of dogmatic atheistic critiques.

32. See Miller and Thorsen, "Spirituality, Religion, and Health," 24b, with reference to William James's famous foundational text for psychology of religion: *The Varieties of Religious Experience: A Study in Human Nature* (orig. 1902; Cambridge, MA: Harvard University Press, 1961).

33. See Miller and Thorsen, "Spirituality, Religion, and Health," 27a; appealing to William James, they cite his view of religion as "feelings, acts, experiences of individual men [*sic*] in their solitude" and then comment, "Thus, in essence, [James] equated religion with spirituality and ignored institutional religion." This approach in turn guides their own view of spirituality.

tercessory *success*.[34] In the light of our complex account of meanings of spiritual healing (above), we may well question whether this is a sufficiently nuanced criterion of actual healing. We can only conclude that such trials on the relation of spirituality and health, while capable of raising some intriguing open questions, hardly scrape the surface either of the theological or scientific intricacies involved; in particular, the rich hermeneutical approaches of both the pray-ers and the pray-ees are deliberately suppressed. The reduction of intercession to a commodified slot-machine model in some prayer studies, combined with what Harrington calls the "eliminative logic" of a straightforward choice between medical efficacy and divine action,[35] beggars the theological imagination, as well as offending, ironically, the sensibilities of the resistant medical secularist. Neither side is satisfied, and with reason.[36]

Our second, and inverse, example (where the interface between religion and medical science involves what I have called a diluted account of the theological, rather than seeking a pure form of it in manifest divine action) is perhaps less obviously problematic to medical practice, but it still raises many unanswered questions for those interested in the workings of spiritual healing. Our example here would be Herbert Benson's much-publicized work at Harvard on the mind-body relation and the physiological benefits of the "relaxation response," a simple form of meditation learned by patients to alleviate symptoms of fear and discomfort during medical protocols.[37] Criticized dismissively over the years by both doctors and religionists, Benson has bravely endured the scorn with good-natured equanimity, and one can but admire his persistence; for there is *no doubt* of the clinical efficacy of taught meditative practice for most patients confronting pain and anxiety in treatments for cancer and other life-threatening ailments. But the criticisms do also have point. For if meditation is reduced to a "relaxation response" and the faith factor generalized as some interchangeable *additum* that remains curiously unanalyzed and homogenized,

34. See Miller and Thorsen, "Spirituality, Religion, and Health," 31a. To be fair, they themselves press, by the end of their article, to a much richer set of themes to be investigated, rather than mere longevity: "Most people want to live with better health, less disease, greater inner peace, and a fuller sense of meaning, direction and satisfaction in their lives" (33b).

35. See again Harrington (chapter 6), p. 129.

36. For a further discerning and wide-ranging assessment of prayer studies (which comes to similar critical conclusions to mine, albeit from a sociological perspective), see Wendy ← Cadge, "Saying Your Prayers, Constructing Your Religions: Medical Studies of Intercessory Prayer," *Journal of Religion* 89 (2009): 299–327.

37. See Herbert Benson, *The Relaxation Response* (New York: Morrow, 1975). The method of meditation taught under this rubric is more akin to what (in Christian terminology) is often termed *acquired contemplation* rather than intellectual or imaginative meditation on a text.

the scientific guild may well wonder at the rigor of the analysis, just as the reli-
gionist or theologian will baulk at the reductivism of theological understanding
involved. There is little cognizance here of the way in which *different* metaphysical commitments and beliefs will profoundly affect the tone (not to speak of the
neurological correlates) of the practices involved; nor is there the least hint of
the possibility that deep and prolonged meditation (or contemplation, as silent
attention to God is termed in the Christian tradition) may over time bring as
much spiritual pain as it dispels — though of a transformed and transforming nature.[38] The point is that investigation of these complexities (which are integral to
the traditions of religious practice involved) again demands *diachronic* narrative
and "hermeneutical" explication; these are not mere physiological *functions* but
meaning-infused practices held through a lifetime of personal transformation.
Any set of scientific explorations that fails to take account of these complexities
is therefore not scientific at all, let alone religiously or theologically profound;
it is, we might say, but a superficial scan of the religiously immature.

The Texture of Theological Accounts of Spiritual Healing

I have allowed myself some harsh comments in the foregoing section about
misbegotten attempts to capture the divine in the nexus of medical investigation, or — contrariwise — to disguise it in some conveniently secularized form
for pragmatic, therapeutic purposes. In both these cases, it has become clear
that the transition to the theological from the medical in questions of spiritual
healing should be seen as a complex and subtle matter, much richer and stranger
indeed than is commonly understood. At least two lessons, I suggest, emerge
from this discussion. The first is that an attentive, sensitive *anthropological* account of spiritual healing (even though, *qua* secular social science, it necessarily
stops short of full-blown theological assessment) provides us with a narrative
bridge between the disciplines of science and theology from which the next step
to sophisticated *metaphysical* speculation and discussion may best take off; for

---

38. Benson has, of course, attempted more than once to respond to some of these criti-
cisms: see Herbert Benson, *Beyond the Relaxation Response: How to Harness the Power of Your
Personal Beliefs* (New York: Times, 1984), and *Timeless Healing: The Power and Biology of Belief*
(New York: Scribner, 1996).

I discuss Benson's work in more detail — both appreciatively and critically — in Sarah
Coakley, "Palliative or Intensification? Pain and Christian Contemplation in the Spiritu-
ality of the Sixteenth Century Carmelites," in *Pain and Its Transformations*, ed. Coakley and
Shelemay, 77–100. See also the discussion and debate with Benson and others in ibid., 133–37.

to ignore the thick description of healing of any sort is to hypothesize vainly, in both medicine and theology.[39] The second lesson, as we shall now discuss, is that the further move to explicitly philosophical and theological reflection about spiritual healing (including theorizing about the nature of the mind/body relation and about purported divine actions and their intersection with the world) is one that itself has no *uncontestable* status: the debate is necessarily an open one. And that applies to secularists and skeptics as much as it does to religious believers. For even those who aver that they have "no need for that [divine] hypothesis" have already made a metaphysical *choice* in favor of naturalism, one that is itself open to debate.[40] The important question, then, is how to adjudicate between the great variety of metaphysical choices on offer.

It falls to Philip Clayton in this volume (chapter 7) to provide a succinct, pointed, and wide-ranging account of how metaphysical issues impinge on the topic of spiritual healing, and of which philosophical and theological models might best attract our attention and respect. Moreover, his contribution follows on from two instructive historical accounts earlier in the book of how we got to this particular metaphysical debate about spiritual healing in the modern and late modern periods. Thus, Emma Anderson's discussion (chapter 2) of Marian apparitions in the late nineteenth century in France highlights how the Roman Catholic authorities' response to them ultimately took on the challenge to claim to *vindicate* their miraculous authenticity, specifically utilizing modern philosophical and medical categories in order to show that, in these cases, they could not apply; whereas, rather differently, but in parallel development, the emergence of Christian Science in New England (and the explosion of other forms of Protestant faith healing at a similar period) manifested — as Heather Curtis shows in chapter 3 — an equally modern desire to highlight the demonstrable importance of the moral, the affective, and the hortatory in explaining the efficacy and fruits of spiritual healing.

---

39. Few social scientists now explain away religious events wholly in terms of other, reductive categories. Thomas Csordas explains his own particular phenomenological method at the start of chapter 9. For more detail on the method of phenomenology as applied within medical anthropology, see Csordas's *The Sacred Self: A Cultural Phenomenology of Charismatic* ⟵ *Healing* (Berkeley: University of California Press, 1994).

40. Of course (as Clayton discusses in his chapter), the initial *presumption* in scientific research is a naturalistic one, but one must distinguish here between methodological and (more metaphysically dogmatic) ontological naturalism. The former does not necessarily imply or require the latter. For a discerning critical discussion of the metaphysics of naturalism, which exposes some of its difficulties, see Michael C. Rea, *World without Design: The* ⟵ *Ontological Consequences of Naturalism* (Oxford: Clarendon, 2002).

Clayton's account of the proper relation (as he sees it) of science, philosophy, and theology to spiritual healing in some ways recapitulates and clarifies these earlier nineteenth-century responses. Like the Protestant healers discussed by Curtis, Clayton prefers to restrict the realm of purported spiritual healings to that of the human *mind* rather than to any interruptions of normal causal processes in the physical body.[41] But unlike the Roman magisterial approach to the miraculous, he avers that it is altogether unwise to attribute to any divine action a status "*separate* from the world, such that it would take a divine incursion into the world in order for God to be associated with inner-worldly happenings."[42] This, he asserts, could only recapitulate the mistake characteristically made in modernity, that of ranging science (or medicine) in straightforward combat with theological claims. For that reason, he himself opts for an "emergentist" view of the human mind, and a "panentheistic" account of divine and human relations: both these metaphysical options, as he sees it, avoid the "eliminative logic" of a direct clash between science and theology. Clayton's overriding concern here is thus to defuse the modernistic war between science and theology, while at the same time granting the methodological naturalism of science and social science an *initial* priority over claims to divine intervention — as more obviously vindicated, he believes, by empirical study.[43] It follows that, for Clayton, metaphysical claims about mind and God can stand only if they take a form that is finally justified by their success in providing the "inference to the best explanation," a criterion of truth that, as he points out, is applied just as demandingly in secular philosophy of science.[44]

Clayton's refreshingly clear account of the *unavoidability* of complex metaphysical debate in relation to claims for spiritual healing seemingly makes no concessions, however, to those who might already hold *prior* theological commitments when discerning the veridicality of such claims. Why is this? After all, there are a number of well-honed approaches to the rationality of religious belief in contemporary philosophy of religion that do not lean on the strong version of justification from empirical evidences and metaphysical arguments

41. See Clayton, p. 152: "it is . . . at the level of human mental causation, that one can most plausibly locate one's account of divine influence in cases of spiritual healing." This move on his part is perhaps unexpected given Clayton's simultaneous rejection of a separatist dualism between mind and body in his "emergentist" theory of the mind.

42. Clayton, p. 150; my emphasis.

43. He gives a lot of ground here to the scientific skeptics; see pp. 134–36, 137–44.

44. The outstanding contemporary analysis of the philosophical status of this "inference" is Peter Lipton, *Inference to the Best Explanation*, 2nd ed. (London: Routledge, 2004).

favored by Clayton.[45] Indeed, it has been a notable feature of the nonfoundationalist turn in recent philosophy of religion to insist that belief in God can itself be properly basic (rather as, for instance, our belief in the reliability of our senses is properly basic) and not therefore subject to empirical verification or corroboration in the way sought by Clayton's model.[46] The discerning reader will therefore notice that John Swinton's closing chapter in this volume, on healing and hermeneutics, does not make any attempt such as Clayton's to justify his (prior) belief in God as a God who heals; he simply assumes that metaphysical hypothesis for the sake of his further explication of the crucial mediating importance of the hermeneutical mode in the experience of those who *are* healed by God.[47]

This important divergence already evident in the theological offerings contained within this volume is highly instructive for those interested in the rationality of the claims made for spiritual healing in the strong, theological sense outlined earlier. For it now becomes clear that a range of possible options confront the specialist in philosophy of religion and theology here, all of them in principle defensible, but via different strategies; and the two we have already noted may be supplemented by a third, which I now outline. Arguably this provides a particularly effective fit with the cumulative picture of spiritual healing that builds in this book — from neuroscience to social science to philosophy of religion and theology. And that is the approach to divine action *through* intercessory prayer and other forms of human cooperation with God's providential purposes that in Western scholastic thought is termed secondary causation. Let me explain further.

In the thought of Thomas Aquinas, this theory of secondary causation is predicated, most importantly, on a vision of divine primary causation as timelessly sustaining the creation in being at every moment and thus providing the underlying matrix for all human *cooperation* (*qua* secondary causation) with God's salvific purposes.[48] Since God's Being is perceived here as "pure

45. For acute, but diverging, accounts of the various meanings of *justification* in modern analytic epistemology, especially as it relates to religious claims, see Richard Swinburne, *Epistemic Justification* (Oxford: Oxford University Press, 2001); and William P. Alston, *Beyond "Justification": Dimensions of Epistemic Evaluation* (Ithaca, NY: Cornell University Press, 2005).

46. See Alvin Plantinga and Nicholas Wolterstorff, eds., *Faith and Rationality: Reason and Belief in God* (Notre Dame: University of Notre Dame Press, 1983), which launched this development in religious epistemology known as Reformed Epistemology.

47. Chapter 10.

48. Thomas Aquinas discusses his understanding of the relation of "primary cause" (*prima causa*) in God and "secondary cause" (*secunda causa*) in creatures in a variety of places in his oeuvre, but see especially *Summa contra gentiles* III, 70, 77, *Summa theologiae* Ia, q. 103 and q. 105, and *Quaestiones disputatae de potentia* 3, 7. Note that, for Aquinas, God's primary

act" (*actus purus*), nothing could be more misleading than the picture often purveyed of Thomas's view of God as somehow frozen and distant in his time-lessness. Moreover, this is a very different picture of the relation of God and the creation from that suggested by Clayton when he objects to what he calls a "dualistic" idea of God as "separate" from the world and thus as needing to make "incursions" into it (from elsewhere, above?) in order to effect acts such as spiritual healing. (To this, his "panentheistic" alternative is presented as a more palatable, convincing, and "immanentist" corrective.) The spatially "separate" notion of the divine to which Clayton objects is indeed very hard to expunge from the Western theistic religious consciousness, for obvious reasons of biblical precedent,[49] and perhaps especially since the modern period when the rise of secular science and philosophy caused some believers to retreat — in reaction — to a deistic notion of God as only occasionally interfering in the world's workings, postcreation.

But the point is that this very picture of spatial separation is what has to be challenged at the outset if a different perception of what might be happening in Christian spiritual healing is to be explicated and embraced according to the scholastic theory of secondary causation. This is a perception, moreover, that is acutely alert to the thick description of how intercessory prayer, restoration to religious community, and positive narrative meaning-making converge in any event of such healing. Such, indeed, was the distinctive nexus of Jesus's own healings, as Beverly Gaventa outlines with such clarity in chapter 1 of this volume. What the gospel healings repeatedly show, in fact, is that Jesus was not simply committed to curing those who sought his healing but to restoring them to self-respect and freedom from guilt and shame, and to reuniting them to a worshiping community and wider society in which they, in turn, would have

---

causal activity is always required (in order for secondary causes to *be* causes) on more than one count: for secondary causes could not do any causing of their own without God, first, creating and preserving them; God giving them, second, the causal powers they have; and God, third, applying the created cause to act. For Aquinas, this last condition does *not* in-volve direct determinism, although he is sometimes misunderstood in this way. What it does involve, however, is an inexorably *paradoxical* notion of the intersection of the timed and the timeless, which greatly complicates the understanding of a divine act: for a famous modern attempt to clarify and resolve this issue, see Eleonore Stump and Norman Kretzmann, "Eter-nity," *Journal of Philosophy* 78 (1981): 429–58. I am grateful to Michael Rota for a number of illuminating conversations on causation in Aquinas.

49. The spatial two-tiered universe generally presumed in the biblical text is, however, not without occasional intimations of a sense of divine timelessness and undergirding suste-nance: see, for example, Pss. 90:1–4; 139:7–10, 17–18; Job 38:4–7; 2 Pet. 3:8; and in relation to Christ: 1 Pet. 1:20; Heb. 13:8; John 17:5; Rev. 1:8.

a future and positive role to play in furthering God's providential plans. In other words, healing is here not simply an extrinsic supernatural intervention into natural events but has a deeper mystery to it in which intercessors, friends, and other members of the body of Christ play their own distinctive and secondary part as mediators and supporters in the ongoing process of healing.

In the theology of Thomas Aquinas, it is this (seemingly paradoxical but absolutely inseparable) juxtaposition of the foundational divine Being and the dependent created order that undergirds Aquinas's vision of the relation of primary and secondary causation, in which God and the world are *never in competition for space*. For on this view, God is precisely *not* another item in the universe (a very big one, in the naive religious mind), who is forced to discern when, or when not, to interfere in a cosmos that is already up and running independently of him. On the contrary, God — if there is a God! — is by definition "that without which there would be nothing at all," that which already wills and loves and holds all created being in existence at all times. That is not, of course, to say that God does *not* also act, specifically and sometimes purely or miraculously in Aquinas's sense,[50] as well as in the continuing divine act of holding us always in being; but it is to say that God's acts, being *God's*, are unlikely to be capable of being itemized and boxed with the simplistic forms of identification that the recent scientific "experiments" on healing have seemed to presume. As we have already noted, bad science and questionable theology tend to go together.

Moreover, this vision of the relation of God to the world coheres closely in Aquinas's thinking with his theory of what is happening in Christian intercessory prayer, such as that offered in a healing service on behalf of others, but also more generally in prayers of petition and intercession.[51] To the obvious objection that, if God is omniscient, omnipotent, and impassible, what possible difference or *additum* could reside in the prayers of others for a suffering one, Thomas's response is again founded in his vision of the church as an extension of Christ's "mystical body": we do not change God's mind in praying for another,

---

50. On Aquinas's view, a miracle is a pure act of God without intermediaries (see *Summa contra gentiles* III, 101, 102; *Summa theologiae* Ia, q. 105, 7), not — as in post-Humean, modern thought — an abrogation of a natural law; see Richard Swinburne's clear exposition of this important difference in *The Concept of Miracle* (London: Macmillan, 1970).

51. *Relation* is a tricky word here, although difficult to avoid altogether; strictly speaking, according to Aquinas, *we* relate to God but not God to *us*, since God is already more intimately (and timelessly) connected to us than this word can adequately convey. See *Summa theologiae* Ia, q. 13, 7: "Now since God is altogether outside the order of creatures, since they are ordered to him but not he to them, it is clear that being related to God is a reality in creatures, but being related to creatures is not a reality in God."

but we do participate thereby more deeply in the propulsion of Christ's suffering, death, and resurrection in our act of love and compassion for the suffering one.[52] It is for that reason that God *wills* us to pray for others and thereby also to participate more deeply in Christ's own salvific work at the level of "secondary causation." There are, of course, necessary and persistent reminders in Aquinas's thought about the extent to which humans in this life can fully grasp the mystery of divine providential purposes and our own cooperative role in them; but it would be a mistake to deride Thomas's negative theology, so-called, as mere mystification. Rather, it is his own disciplined way of insisting that *any* speculation about God is attended by a necessary stammering in the face of Being itself; even Thomas's famous arguments for God's existence end with the reminder that the acknowledgment of the force of these arguments must be held alongside the profound sensibility of his ultimate unknowability.[53]

To conclude, one of the important outcomes from these theological reflections on healing, and the metaphysical choices presented to us in them, is that the matter of God's *existence* is unlikely to be settled by appeal to the evidence of purported spiritual healings *alone*. Even Philip Clayton's strong justificatory approach acknowledges that point, to the extent that he rightly draws attention to major metaphysical debates and choices that must be confronted in debates about healing, *prior* to any final adjudication of the best explanation of such events. The decision for or against the rationality of religious belief, therefore, is a matter that at some point will probably engage the issue of healing; but to make purported healings bear the full load of such an assent would be to risk turning them into what the Gospel of John (at points disparagingly) calls "signs."[54] The point here, to repeat, is that an authentic Christian healing is not

52. Brian Davies, OP, "God and Prayer," in his *Thinking About God* (Eugene, OR: Wipf & Stock, 2010), 307–33, provides an exemplary account of the philosophical problems of intercessory prayer to an impassible God, and he offers a convincing exposition of Aquinas's response. For a more critical, analytic assessment of Aquinas's position on prayer, see Eleonore Stump, "Petitionary Prayer," *American Philosophical Quarterly* 16 (1979): 81–91.

53. See *Summa theologiae* Ia, q. 2, 3, which ends, "Now we cannot know what God is, but only what he is not" (see also *Summa contra gentiles* I, 14). Fergus Kerr, OP, comments, in his *After Aquinas: Versions of Thomism* (Oxford: Blackwell, 2002), 58: "From the start, the 'theistic proofs' are the first lesson in Thomas's negative theology. Far from being an exercise in rationalistic apologetics, the purpose of arguing for God's existence is to protect God's transcendence."

54. Beverly Roberts Gaventa discusses John's theology of signs briefly in chapter 1 (see pp. 34 and 38). On the one hand, the major miraculous signs in John's Gospel are authentic indications of Jesus's messianic status (John 7:31); but to the extent that people seek him out merely for such signs as extrinsic performances, John makes it clear that there is a much

one that merely effects an extrinsic cure (although that may well also be the case) but one that has wider spiritual and moral effects of transformation, for the healers as well as the one healed.[55]

Spiritual Healing in Pastoral Perspective

What follows, then, from our theological discussion of *metaphysical* options in the explanation of spiritual healing is a final, and crowning, reflection on how the nexus of interdisciplinary insights gathered in this volume might play out in pastoral practice.

Especially since the charismatic renewal in the latter part of the twentieth century, expectations of spiritual healing in Christian circles have both dramatically reintensified and yet also gradually become more routinized, according to ecclesiastical context.[56] The more dramatic forms of healing described by Thomas Csordas (chapter 9) continue, of course, in charismatic and Pentecostal circles worldwide; but practices of this sort are also now commonly found in quieter and more formalized healing rituals in most mainline Christian denominations in the West. Such, indeed, has been the remarkable long-term cultural and ecclesiastical impact of the earlier charismatic renewal, that spiritual healing in some form or another is now an expectation rather than an exception in both Protestant and Catholic churches. I am assuming that at least some of the readers of this book will be ministers and laity engaged in such parish practices of healing; and my sincere hope is that this volume will assist them in thinking through the complex intersection of scientific, medical, philosophical, and theological issues that these undertakings necessarily represent.

The theological and pastoral danger in the current popularity of such rituals

---

deeper level of response to him that is required in true faith (see John 12:37-38; 2:23-25). Note also that even contemporary philosophers of religion who still wish to make miracles part of an empirical argument for God's existence characteristically do not claim that such an appeal *on its own* could sway the case; see Richard Swinburne, *The Existence of God*, 2nd ed. (Oxford: Clarendon, 2004), ch. 12, who argues that purported miracles may represent one element in a complex "cumulative case" for God's existence.

55. See Beverly Roberts Gaventa (chapter 1) and John Swinton (chapter 10) for more extensive reflections on this point, and Stephen Clark (chapter 8) for a rather different focus on the *moral* discernment involved in healing.

56. The classic overview of the history of healing in the Christian churches remains Morton T. Kelsey, *Healing and Christianity: A Classic Study*, 3rd ed. (orig. 1973; Minneapolis: Augsburg Fortress, 1995), which brings the story up to include the later effects on mainstream denominations of the charismatic renewal.

across the denominations, however, is perhaps not so much that they intensify the theodicy question about why God chooses to heal some and not others (a question sensitively responded to in John Swinton's chapter in this book), but rather that the rituals involved can easily become mechanical, repetitive, and even talismanic, divorced both from well-informed *theological* teaching about healing and from the context of deep and trusting prayer that — as Christian healers of significant reputation aver — opens the space for God to be God in those who call on him. As those experienced in this ministry testify, any false manipulation of power in this context is an immediate sign of something being awry; any genuine manifestation of the "fruits of the Spirit" (Gal. 5:22–26) is a sure indication of divine confirmation. Healing in its authentic forms, then, always involves a narrative embedded in a realm of moral and religious meaning, and should be founded in spiritual practices of some depth and demand for those exercising ministry in this area.[57]

What the essays in this volume cumulatively suggest in relation to the pastoral context of healing, I believe, are at least the following lessons for pastoral practice:

1. The meaning-making context (biblical and theological teaching, bodily prayer and liturgical spiritual practices, social and community relations of trust) is all-important in any event of healing; this fact may not be explicitly or consciously expressed at the time of the healing rite itself, but it informs all that happens and requires careful thinking and regular review. If healing rituals become dislocated from such hermeneutics (in the wide sense explored in detail in this book), they can easily slide toward superstitious repetitions or expectations of extrinsic magic.

2. Prayerful preparation and attentiveness to the mood and desires of a suffering individual by those engaged in the healing practices (as all the thick-description examples in this book demonstrate) are equally significant in efficacious rites of healing, as is strict professionalism in the keeping of confidences. Healing cannot be forced on anyone who does not ask for it;[58] the danger here nowadays is often in a formulaic or overly quick imposition of certain newly retrieved ancient practices (laying on

57. Stephen Parsons's *The Challenge of Christian Healing* (London: SPCK, 1986) remains one of the wisest and most discerning pastoral accounts of gifted healers and their practices in the parish context.

58. Recall, as does Beverly Gaventa in chapter 1, the importance in Jesus's healings of the motivational desire and faith of the suffering person (or the one interceding for him or her); see, for example, Mark 9:24; Luke 7:9; John 5:6.

of hands, anointing, confession: see James 5:13–16) at a moment that may not be right for the suffering person. Prayerfulness, patience, gentleness, and a nonjudgmental attitude are crucial in the discernment of meaning involved in any passage to healing. Theologically speaking, these are the accompanying signs of the efficacious secondary causation that leans on God's primary and ever-present sustenance.

3. Background teaching and critical thinking about scientific, medical, and philosophical issues in relation to spiritual healing are also, I submit, more important than is usually acknowledged in the parochial context. Any parish will contain at least some people who are initially skeptical about healing practices, because they wish to think through the relation between what is claimed for such practices and what is offered by clinical medicine and scientific explanation in comparison. Others, perhaps less skeptical, will nonetheless welcome the chance to reflect on the profound theological and philosophical issues that are raised by prayers for healing. Sensitive and well-informed teaching in these areas is thus an invaluable background accompaniment to the healing practices themselves and need in no way abrogate the mysterious and prayerful nature of the interactions of healing itself. But it will also in some important respects (indirectly) affect the tenor of the healing rite, the attitude and expectations of the healers, and the care of the suffering person. For the crucial questions always press implicitly on that person, at the moment of acutest distress: should she accept each and every medical treatment offered? Is all her hope for recovery founded in the scientific or medical world? What exactly is she expecting of God, in contrast? This book has been designed to help with various dimensions of these big questions.

4. The most profound healing at the end of life may well come with the acceptance of death in the face of a medical megalith that often refuses and denies it; if so, the meaning one has made of one's life in relation to God will here reach its greatest crisis and final climax. Preparing for this eventuality earlier in life, difficult as this is, is thus what is crucially important in the spiritual development of all Christians and, in particular, should be part of the theological training of all those involved in any serious commitment to spiritual healing. In short, theological training in *memento mori* is an unavoidable part of the final *ars moriendi*.[59]

---

59. Although he does not employ these traditional Christian terms, Atul Gawande faces these issues of end-of-life preparation and acceptance of death with remarkable sensitivity and insight in his bestselling book *Being Mortal: Illness, Medicine, and What Matters in the End*

We return, therefore, at the end of this introduction, to the core themes with which we opened it. In the context of the Western cultural contradictions over health and suffering that we have explored at some length in this introduction, the phenomenon of spiritual healing is at base a manifestation that calls forth a world of *value*. The question for any sufferer, therefore, is *what* values are finally at stake; and despite all the mystery that enshrines any event of spiritual healing we may encounter, this is a question that requires the taking of thought at many different levels of reflection. This book is designed to help the reader in that quest.

Editor's note: The final proofs for this volume were reviewed in June/July 2020, during the COVID-19 pandemic and the national demonstrations in the United States against racial injustice. The subject of the hermeneutics of healing and the (related) hermeneutics of injustice seems now more pressing than ever; and the editor hopes and prays that this book may contribute in some small way to ameliorative reflection on what deeply troubles this nation and the world about us.

— *SC*

(London: Profile, 2015). I return to Gawande's personal narrative briefly at the opening of my conclusion to this book, below.

Part One

Biblical and Historical Perspectives

I

Healing, Meaning, and Discernment
in the Biblical Text

Beverly Roberts Gaventa

W hat is the meaning of healing in the Bible? This question turns out to disclose some more profound and subtle issues than might be presumed. Contemporary readers of the Bible often find themselves both drawn to and mystified by accounts of spiritual healings and see them as miracles in which God or some agent of God performs a special act that cures an afflicted individual of some disease or debilitating condition. But this way of reading the biblical accounts severely distorts their depiction of spiritual healing, which is but one strand intricately woven into the vast biblical story of God's creation and redemption of humanity. Spiritual healing in the Bible extends well beyond the correction of an individual's problem and is deeply embedded in human communities that are themselves restored and empowered by healing. Further, spiritual healing is the subject of a process of discernment about the source and meaning of the healing itself.

Biblical Stories of Healing: A Textured Phenomenon

Now Simon's mother-in-law was in bed with a fever, and they told [Jesus] about her at once. He came and took her by the hand and lifted her up. Then the fever left her, and she began to serve them. (Mark 1:30–31)[1]

1. All biblical quotations are from the New Revised Standard Version, unless otherwise noted.

This simple, direct account takes place in the opening chapter of the Gospel of Mark, widely regarded as the earliest of the Gospels. Many biblical accounts of spiritual healing give the impression, at least at first glance, of being similarly straightforward. Jesus encounters a leper who asks for healing and receives it (Mark 1:40–44; cf. Matt. 8:1–4; Luke 5:12–16). A woman who has suffered from a crippling condition for eighteen years is restored to health when Jesus pronounces her healed and lays hands on her (Luke 13:10–17). With the words, "Lazarus, come out," Jesus restores life to a man who has been dead for four days (John 11:1–44).

Such simple presentations of spiritual healing are both alien from and appealing to contemporary readers, perhaps especially those in the West. The hemorrhaging woman whom Jesus heals (Mark 5:24b–34) does not need to consider whether to pursue biomedical treatment or alternative therapies, does not question whether the treatment will be appropriate and effective, and does not find herself rambling in a maze of telephone calls and paperwork. She merely finds herself in the presence of the Healer and goes away restored. Small wonder that the church's preachers and teachers so often hear the question, "Why isn't that sort of healing taking place now, for me, for my loved one, for my friend?"

Before dismissing these scriptural healing accounts as hopelessly irrelevant to the matters addressed by other essays in this volume, it is important to understand that biblical perspectives on healing are far more complex than is apparent in the account of any single incident. In biblical literature, spiritual healing is a richly textured phenomenon. A first indication of the complexity of spiritual healing in biblical perspective is the sheer range of events involved. As noted above, what comes to mind initially are occasions when people are healed of physical ailments. The Gospels relate many situations in which Jesus performs healings, including the healing of paralysis, leprosy, hemorrhage, blindness, and even death itself. Indeed, one dominant thread in the Gospels' presentation of Jesus is that of healer.[2]

---

2. In addition to treatments of individual stories in commentaries, see the following works devoted to healing: Alan Richardson, *The Miracle Stories of the Gospel* (New York: Harper & Row, 1941); Reginald Fuller, *Interpreting the Miracles* (London: SCM, 1963); Hendrik Van der Loos, *The Miracles of Jesus* (Leiden: Brill, 1965); Morton T. Kelsey, *Healing and Christianity in Ancient Thought and Modern Times* (New York: Harper & Row, 1973); Gerd Theissen, *The Miracle Stories of the Early Christian Tradition* (Philadelphia: Fortress, 1983); Stevan L. Davies, *Jesus the Healer: Possession, Trance, and the Origins of Christianity* (New York: Continuum, 1995); John Pilch, *Healing in the New Testament: Insights from Medical and Mediterranean Anthropology* (Minneapolis: Fortress, 2000).

Yet spiritual healings are not performed by Jesus alone. Prominent among Old Testament healings are the stories of Elijah's healing of Naaman's leprosy and his restoration of life to the son of the widow of Zarephath (1 Kings 17:17–24; a similar healing is attributed to Elisha in 2 Kings 4:18–37). In addition, the Acts of the Apostles recounts healings brought about through the agency of the apostles. Peter and John heal a man who has been crippled from his birth (Acts 3:1–10), and Peter heals a man suffering from paralysis and restores life to the dead disciple Tabitha (9:32–43). Paul also heals a man crippled from birth (Acts 13:8–18); later Luke reports that handkerchiefs that had touched Paul's skin had healing properties (Acts 19:12; and see 28:7–10).

Most of these healings are concerned with conditions or ailments that are readily understandable to modern readers, but several variations in biblical healings press the boundaries of what is normally regarded as matters of illness. Prominent among Jesus's healings is the act of exorcism, a condition that involves neither disease nor birth defect, but conflict with the demonic.[3] A typical story of exorcism is the following:

> Just then there was in the synagogue a man with an unclean spirit, and he cried out, "What have you to do with us, Jesus of Nazareth? Have you come to destroy us? I know who you are, the Holy One of God." But Jesus rebuked him, saying, "Be silent, and come out of him!" And the unclean spirit, convulsing him and crying with a loud voice, came out of him. They were all amazed, and they kept on asking one another, "What is this? A new teaching — with authority! He commands even the unclean spirits, and they obey him." At once his fame began to spread throughout the surrounding region of Galilee. (Mark 1:23–28)

By contrast with the first group of healings, in which the healer addresses the afflicted individual directly, in this instance, the healer addresses the unclean spirit. And the spirit resists, unwilling to give up its power over the man. Although biblical narratives elsewhere present illness as part of the natural course of things, as in the woman with a fever or the woman with a hemorrhage, here the stories are of conflict between divine power and the powers that resist God. Acts 16 provides an elegant twist to this motif: Paul exorcises from an unnamed

---

3. On exorcism in the New Testament, see Vernon McCasland, *By the Finger of God* (New York: Macmillan, 1951); Graham H. Twelftree, *Jesus the Exorcist* (Tübingen: Mohr Siebeck, 1993); John Christopher Thomas, *The Devil, Disease and Deliverance: Origins of Illness in New Testament Thought*, Journal of Pentecostal Theology Supplement Series 13 (Sheffield: Sheffield Academic, 1998).

slave woman a demon that led her to tell fortunes and thereby to enrich her owners, and the exorcism places Paul in conflict not only with the demon but with the enraged owners who have now lost a source of income.[4]

The element of conflict is particularly vivid in Mark 5, which opens with an extensive description of the powerlessness of the afflicted man. He is no longer part of the human community, having been so dominated by the demon that he cannot be subdued, and is reduced to living alongside the dead, howling aloud and even inflicting pain on himself. As in the instance mentioned above in Mark 1, Jesus confronts the demon directly and gains access to its name, "Legion." At the demon's request, Jesus sends it into a herd of swine, which Legion then so completely controls that they are plunged down a bank and into the sea. Other exorcisms likewise underscore this element of conflict between Jesus and demonic powers (for example, Mark 9:14–29).

Numerous biblical stories of miraculous births may also be regarded as spiritual healings, although they are not customarily treated as such.[5] Several important points in Israel's history are marked by accounts of births to women who have long been unable to conceive. The best-known and most influential of these stories is that of Sarah, who, according to the biblical narrative, gives birth to her son Isaac only after her ninetieth birthday (Gen. 17:17). Other barren women who give birth include the women of Abimelech's household (Gen. 20:17–18), Rebekah (Gen. 25:21), Rachel (Gen. 30:22–24), the unnamed wife of Manoah, mother of Samson (Judg. 13:2–3), and Hannah, mother of Samuel (1 Sam. 1:1–20). Luke's Gospel closely follows these accounts of barrenness and birth in the story of the birth of John the Baptist to Elizabeth and Zechariah (Luke 1:8–25). These traditional accounts of healing barren women are replayed with a dramatic twist in the story of Mary's conception, in which the young and unmarried Mary conceives without a human partner (Luke 1:26–38).

To be sure, these events are rarely labeled as healings, although Genesis 20:17–18 explicitly states that "God healed Abimelech, and also healed his wife and female slaves so that they bore children." The role of God in such stories is expressed in various ways, as in Genesis 21:1, where the text asserts that "The Lord dealt with Sarah as he had said, and the Lord did for Sarah as he had promised." Rebekah's conception occurs because the Lord grants the prayer of Isaac (Gen. 25:21), Rachel's because "God remembered" and "heeded her and opened her womb" (Gen. 30:22), and an angel of the Lord foretells Samson's birth (Judg.

4. On this and other exorcisms in Luke-Acts, see Todd Klutz, *The Exorcism Stories in Luke-Acts* (Cambridge: Cambridge University Press, 2004).

5. The question whether barrenness is understood as an illness in ancient medical tradition and in Luke-Acts is taken up by Annette Weissenrieder, *Images of Illness in the Gospel of Luke* (Tübingen: Mohr Siebeck, 2003), 76–100.

13:2–24). The role of God in these conceptions is celebrated in Psalm 113:9: "He gives the barren woman a home, / making her the joyous mother of children." Such exultation rings particularly true in a culture that attached overwhelming significance to childbearing and regarded the childless woman with disdain. It is easy to understand why Rachel responds to her conception, "God has taken away my reproach" (Gen. 30:24), and why Elizabeth says that God "took away the disgrace I have endured among my people" (Luke 1:25). In this society, reproductive health and social standing were thoroughly intertwined.

Yet another complexity in the biblical treatment of spiritual healing is that healing takes place in the context of stories of punishment and restoration. Stories of barren women who finally are able to conceive may assume that the barrenness is a sign of divine displeasure, as in Genesis 20:17–18 (cited above). When Miriam and Aaron question Moses's leadership, God becomes angry with them and Miriam becomes leprous, only to be restored to health after the intervention of both Aaron and Moses (Num. 12:1–16). In a later episode, the grumbling of the Israelites in the desert provokes God, who sends poisonous serpents as a punishment and later (after Moses again intercedes) provides for healing (Num. 21:4–9). Similarly, King Jeroboam's hand is withered as a punishment and restored only after prayer on his behalf (1 Kings 13:1–10). The motif of punishment and restoration may also be at work in the story of Acts 9, in which Saul's encounter with the risen Jesus leaves him blind, to be restored to sight only after the visit of Ananias.

These varying stories come together in the identification of God as the healer of Israel. The declaration that "I am the Lord who heals you" (Exod. 15:26) is frequently reaffirmed in the Old Testament:

> See now that I, even I, am he; there is no god besides me. I kill and I make alive; I wound and I heal; and no one can deliver from my hand. (Deut. 32:39)

> I have seen their ways, but I will heal them; I will lead them and repay them with comfort, creating for their mourners the fruit of the lips. Peace, peace, to the far and the near, says the LORD; and I will heal them. (Isa. 57:18–19)

> For I will restore health to you, and your wounds I will heal, says the LORD. (Jer. 30:17)

The identification of God as the healer of Israel is taken up in the New Testament in descriptions of Jesus as a healer. This is announced dramatically when John the Baptist sends his own disciples to ask whether Jesus is the awaited Messiah, and Jesus responds, "Go and tell John what you have seen and heard:

the blind receive their sight, the lame walk, the lepers are cleansed, the deaf hear, the dead are raised, and the poor have good news brought to them" (Luke 7:22). When asked to explain who he is, Jesus responds in the language of healing. The Fourth Gospel intensifies this identification by labeling Jesus's healings (and other miracles, see John 2:1–12) as "signs" that reveal Jesus's "glory" (for example, 4:54; 6:2; 9:16; 20:30).

Healing and Community

That God is Israel's healer and that Jesus's identity is to be perceived by means of his healings already suggest that spiritual healing in the Bible is not simply a matter of repairing the afflictions and diseases endured by a series of individuals. Healing is integrally involved with community — whether that community be a small local gathering or the whole of Israel. Indeed, the community's role in the phenomenon of spiritual healing is far more extensive than might be imagined simply by noticing the presence of crowds as witnesses in the Gospel stories of Jesus's healing. In fact, the community is itself deeply implicated in the biblical phenomenon of spiritual healing, as will be shown.

In many instances, it is the community's initiative that sets a healing in motion: the community brings its afflicted to Jesus, confident that healing comes from him. The lively story of Jesus's healing of a paralytic opens with the vivid depiction of a group of people digging a hole through a roof in order to place their friend in the presence of Jesus (Mark 2:1–12; cf. Matt. 9:2–8; Luke 5:17–26). On this occasion, Jesus explicitly acknowledges that those who bring the afflicted man have "faith" or "confidence" that he will be healed.[6] In the case of a son of a Roman centurion, someone whom readers would know to be an outsider possibly resented by the local inhabitants, Luke reports that the centurion sends Jewish elders to seek Jesus's help, which prompts Jesus to praise the faith of the centurion (Luke 7:1–10). Elsewhere that faith or confidence in Jesus is tacitly expressed in the very action of bringing a loved one to Jesus, as in Mark 7:31–37, when a man who is able neither to hear nor speak is brought to Jesus by others who "begged him to lay his hand on him" (v. 32; see also Mark 8:22). Occasionally, the Gospels simply summarize Jesus's activity in a particular region, and typically such summaries include reports about local residents who bring their

6. The Greek word *pistis* is conventionally translated as "faith," which in English routinely refers to belief, but it also has connotations of confidence or trust. When Jesus affirms the "faith" of those who come to him, these notions of confidence or trust are involved.

sick to Jesus, as in Mark 6:54b–55: "People at once recognized him, and rushed about that whole region and began to bring the sick on mats to wherever they heard he was" (see also Matt. 4:23–25; 8:16; 14:34–36). The anonymous "they" in these incidents does not require further identification, as the stories serve not to identify and characterize these participants but to make clear that Jesus's power to heal is widely known in communities small and large.

Yet the community is more than a literary device for instigating the healing. The community also stands on the other side of the healing account, providing a witness to and interpretation of the event. In response to the healing of the paralytic, for example, Luke reports that "Amazement seized all of them, and they glorified God and were filled with awe, saying, 'We have seen strange things today'" (Luke 5:26). Following the raising of the widow's son, the crowd is reported to be afraid: "And they glorified God, saying, 'A great prophet has risen among us!' and 'God has looked favorably on his people!'" (Luke 7:16). Similarly, when Peter heals the man at the Jerusalem temple, the crowd is said to be "filled with wonder and amazement."

Such doxologies are not to be understood as signaling universal acceptance and approbation of Jesus's actions and his implied authority, however. It may be that "all the people" "praised God" when they saw the healing of the blind man (Luke 18:43), but in other situations, healing can be disconcerting or controversial. When Jesus heals a woman in a synagogue on the Sabbath, the synagogue leader objects that Jesus has violated Sabbath law (Luke 13:10–17; see also John 5:1–18), and elsewhere, religious leaders characterize Jesus's exorcisms as actions of "the ruler of the demons" (Matt. 9:34). These comments sometimes issue into debates, as in the extended account in John 9, involving the healed man, his parents, "the Jews," and Jesus himself. Another debate of sorts follows upon the healing of the man in the temple precinct by Peter and John; in response to the crowd's amazement, Peter preaches a sermon, following which he and John are arrested for the first time (Acts 3). In the most extreme accounts, Jesus's actions prompt his opponents to conspire to bring about his death (Mark 3:1–6).

Such conflicting responses to Jesus's healings should not obscure the fact that the healings often carry with them the restoration of community, although the restoration is more often implicit rather than explicit. For example, following his healing of a leper, Jesus instructs the man to go to the priest and make the required offering (Mark 1:40–45; see also Luke 17:11–19). This offering is stipulated in Leviticus 14, by way of declaring the individual clean, reversing the earlier declaration that the individual who is leprous "shall live alone; his dwelling shall be outside the camp" (Lev. 13:46); having made the offering, the healed man is able to return to the community. A similar possibility for restoration is involved in the story of the woman suffering from a hemorrhage, since she and everything with which she comes in contact would be rendered ritually impure because of her discharge (at least according to Levitical regulation; see Lev. 15:25–30). The exorcisms also imply release from social isolation, since the stories frequently depict those possessed by demons as utterly out of control. In the story of Legion, the man is reduced to living among the tombs (Mark 5:1–20). Another exorcism, that of a father's only child, concludes with Jesus returning the son to his father, signaling his restoration to the family (Luke 9:37–43). In all these instances, healing is inextricably connected to a wider community or network of relations.

Restoration after healing is, however, not restricted to these situations in which the ritual purity code or demon possession ruptures the community. In a particularly poignant scene, Acts 9 depicts those who mourn for the disciple Tabitha, who had been involved in providing clothing for the widows of Joppa. This loss is overturned by her healing, and her restoration becomes explicit when Peter calls in the mourners so that they see her alive again (9:41). Again, the community context is vital to the significance of the event.

The community's role can also extend beyond that of witnessing and receiving. In some instances, the community itself takes on the more active role, becoming the agent of healing. As noted earlier, the Acts of the Apostles narrates numerous healings accomplished through the agency of Peter and Paul, who, although they are individually named, stand as representatives for believers. It might be objected that Peter and Paul are exceptions, as they are in some sense Jesus's successors rather than representatives of the community at large; but elsewhere, New Testament writers assume that healing is a natural part of the work of the Christian community. In 1 Corinthians 12, as Paul discusses the body of Christ and enumerates the diverse gifts that constitute the one body, he includes healing alongside the work of the apostles, prophets, and teachers (1 Cor. 12:9, 28). The Epistle of James also appears to take this feature of community life for granted, since it exhorts:

> Are any among you sick? They should call for the elders of the church and have them pray over them, anointing them with oil in the name of the Lord. The prayer of faith will save the sick, and the Lord will raise them up; and anyone who has committed sins will be forgiven. (James 5:14–15)

These diverse strands of the New Testament share the same audacious claim that spiritual healing is located within the believing community and is an expected part of it.

Healing and Discernment

In yet another way, biblical stories of healing are a complex phenomenon that transcends the simple curing of an individual. Not only do they involve a range of situations that contemporary readers might not recognize as healing, and in which the community takes part in complex ways, but biblical stories of healing are also often the subject of a complicated process of discernment. Contemporary readers ask whether the healing is real, but ancient readers are far more inclined to ask whose power is involved. The ancient world took for granted the possibility of spiritual healings, as is evidenced in the cult of Asclepius and elsewhere.[7] Overwhelmingly in the Gospels, the question is not the contemporary one of whether a healing is real, but where it comes from: Whose power accomplished the healing, and what does it signify?

The question of whose power is at work in spiritual healings comes into focus sharply when some Pharisees charge that Jesus works by demonic power rather than the power of God. In Matthew 12, the report of Jesus's exorcism brings the charge: "It is only by Beelzebul, the ruler of the demons, that this fellow casts out the demons" (12:24; see also 9:34 par.). This charge prompts Jesus to make the wily observation that an exorcism brought about by Satan effectively pits Satan against himself, since Satan is then casting out his own ally (12:26). The exchange works only because it is assumed that there are several powers capable of exorcism, of healing; the question, then, is whose power is at work.

That question is crucial to the story of Acts 3. When confronted by a man born with a crippling condition, Peter declares: "in the name of Jesus Christ of Nazareth, stand up and walk" (3:6). This invoking of Jesus's name becomes central in the conflict that ensues, for Peter must explain to the bystanders what he means by calling on the name of Jesus (3:11–26). Arrested following their preaching, Peter and John are confronted by the religious authorities who ask, "By what power or by what name did you do this?" (4:7).

There are, to be sure, occasions when invoking the name of Jesus is not effective, making it clear that the act of calling on Jesus's name is not sufficient for healing in some mechanistic way. Apart from faith, calling on Jesus's name can be disastrous, as in the case of the exorcists in Acts 19, who attempt to make use of Jesus's name for their own work. The evil spirit, confronted with a fraudulent

7. Some examples may be found conveniently in Frederick C. Grant, ed., *Hellenistic Religions: The Age of Syncretism* (New York: Liberal Arts, 1953), 49–59; Francis Martin, ed., *Narrative Parallels to the New Testament* (Atlanta: Scholars Press, 1988). And see the helpful discussion of "miracles and ancient minds" in John P. Meier, *A Marginal Jew: Rethinking the Historical Jesus*, vol. 2: *Mentor, Message, and Miracles* (New York: Doubleday, 1994), 535–616.

invocation of Jesus's name, responds, "Jesus I know, and Paul I know, but who are you?" (Acts 19:15). Not only is the exorcism ineffective in this case, but also the pitiful demoniac triumphs over the exorcists, forcing them to retreat without even the dignity of their clothing (19:16). It is not only competing figures who are rendered ineffective, however. Even the disciples themselves sometimes encounter difficulty; although they are reported to cast out demons and to heal the sick (Mark 6:13), there are demons able to resist them, demons who respond only to Jesus (Mark 9:14–29).

Because it is the subject of such discernment, spiritual healing can be misunderstood in a variety of ways. In one scene in Acts, those who witness a healing do not ask whose power is involved; instead, they jump to the erroneous conclusion that Paul's healing of a man who is disabled means that Paul himself is a god in human form, and they summon the local priest to offer sacrifice to Paul and his companion Barnabas, comically misidentified as Hermes and Zeus (14:8–18). Here the response to healing is faith, but faith in the wrong god. John's Gospel offers a more complex presentation of the relationship between spiritual healing (Jesus's "signs") and faith; Jesus's signs ought to evoke faith (2:23–25; 12:37; 20:30–31), but sometimes they evoke only the demand for more such performances (6:2, 26, 30).

Discerning the power that heals and discerning the community's relationship with that power is not an isolated issue for the believing community. In what is widely thought to be the earliest Christian writing, 1 Thessalonians, Paul addresses another spiritual gift, the gift of prophecy. There he instructs the fledgling Christian community not to "quench the Spirit" and not to "despise the words of prophets" (5:19–20), perhaps because certain prophetic excesses had created problems. He continues with the admonition: "test everything; hold fast to what is good; abstain from every form of evil." Prophetic statements are not to be accepted at face value but must be subjected to the scrutiny of the community, so that what is upbuilding (properly affirming of the community, and truly prophetic) is retained and what is destructive is avoided. The same scrutiny presumably applies to the gift of healing, which must be examined not only to discern whether healing is genuine but also whether it is genuinely of God.

That feature of discerning what healing means shifts the discussion again to the larger biblical context of spiritual healing and offers a pointed reminder: in the Bible, spiritual healings are not commodities at the disposal of human agents. They are not even commodities for the repair of individual lives, however laudable such repair may be. Instead, healing has to do with God's will for human flourishing, with the reclamation of all of creation (Rom. 8). As Jesus responds to his critics: "If it is by the Spirit of God that I cast out demons, then the kingdom of God has come to you" (Matt. 12:28).

Conclusion

We began with the simple story in Mark 1, in which Jesus heals Peter's mother-in-law of a fever, a story that could, if taken out of its larger literary and canonical setting, reinforce contemporary notions of miracles as isolated events in which an individual is instantly rescued from an illness or debilitating condition. Certainly miraculous and unexpected events can occur in the biblical narrative. Yet we have seen that healing in the Bible, properly understood, is anything but an isolated and extrinsic phenomenon. It is, rather, integrally related to the larger biblical story of God's creation and restoration of humankind. As such, it takes place in the context of human communities of nurture and faith. And it requires discernment and interpretation within and beyond those communities.

*   *   *

Much of the rest of this book will be taken up with assessing what such discernment and interpretation in relation to spiritual healing should now mean in the contemporary period. But since a marked new skepticism about the "miraculous," *tout court*, was such a striking feature of the modern period, it will be revealing first, by way of immediate background, to turn to two contrasting accounts of spiritual healing in the nineteenth century, in which skeptical scientific reduction was firmly resisted. One account concerns Catholic healings in France; the other, Protestant healings in North America. Both the differences and the commonalities in these stories bespeak their cultural contexts and will provide telling points of comparison with the contemporary scientific and ethnographic material that follows. In all cases, as we shall see, the issue of contextual and community *interpretation* remains vital. In that feature, these narratives are true heirs of the biblical materials just discussed.

2

Healing and Ecclesial Response in
Nineteenth-Century Catholic France

Emma Anderson

This chapter is concerned with certain extraordinary visions and healings received in Catholic Europe in the nineteenth century, and with the contestations about their meaning at different levels of reflection, both popular and official. As will emerge in the telling, much can be learned here about the phenomenon and meaning of spiritual healing in the period of late modernity, as it was presented both interpersonally and ecclesiastically.

The religious experiences of invalids visiting nineteenth-century Marian shrines reflected their strong sense of proximity to a palpable, sacred presence. Testimony of the ill or injured and their families suggests their vivid sense of intimate encounter with a holy immanence, which palpably affected the invalids' perception of their somatic and social circumstances. Invalids' sense of a personal, physical connection to a living divine reality represented their absorption and ratification of the dramatic incidents that had led to the founding of these sites. From the often vague accounts children or adolescents gave of their ambiguous experiences with a lady or a light, Catholic communities in the nineteenth century developed and ritually expressed their belief that the soil, air, and water of the apparition site, sanctified by Mary's presence, had been permeated with thaumaturgical possibility. Through the process of popular interpretation, Mary's reported messages were often eclipsed by popular perceptions of her lingering accessibility, transforming sometimes dire prophetic warnings of the reality of sin and the necessity of repentance into a promise of physical and spiritual redemption. Marian cures, then, represented both a ratification of the apparition sequences, which had founded the shrines, and their subtle reinterpretation along more thaumaturgical lines.

Invalids at Marian healing sites created and challenged established meanings not only in conjunction with Marian seers, with whom, on an experiential level, they shared much in common, but also in contrast with the upper echelons of the Roman Catholic Church, which sought simultaneously to defy and to court the forces of modernity and secularism. In contrast with the more pastoral concerns of parish priests, the higher rungs of the hierarchy were determined to utilize Marian healings to demonstrate the undeniable reality of miraculous, supernatural intervention to skeptics. The attempts of the Catholic hierarchy to convince the medical community of the veracity of Marian miracles eventually led them to adopt the same rigorous standards of proof and evidence as their antagonists and to ignore the broader, more multivalent sense of the miraculous often experienced and expressed by devout lay Catholics. Then, as now, only a tiny fraction of the sick or injured who sought cure at Lourdes or other Marian sites experienced the dramatic alleviation of their physical symptoms. But many of those who did not receive a somatic cure reported experiencing a powerful affirmation of their religious faith, which enabled them, as individuals and families, to face the continued challenges of their lives with renewed vigor, faith, and determination. In their insistence upon the reality of Mary's continuing physical presence at the apparition site, and the beneficial devotional and somatic effects of encountering her there, the Catholic faithful were articulating a wider sense of the miraculous than were the ecclesiastical hierarchy who presumed spiritually to guide them.

Miraculous cures attributed to the maternal intercession of the Virgin Mary in nineteenth-century Europe, then, were the result of a complex process of meaning-negotiation between disparate individuals and groups and were predicated upon a particular interpretation of the apparition events that had founded the shrines: one that emphasized the reality of Mary's ongoing physical presence and its dramatic curative potential. Pivotal events in the private lives of individual invalids, the social and somatic results of spectacular Marian healings came to be critical evidence in the public articulation of contested, contrasting understandings of the relationship between body and soul, sacred and profane, and religion and modernity in the latter half of the nineteenth century. This essay will explore popular and clerical responses to Marian apparitions and healings, and also the process whereby the anomalous experiences of children and adolescents became transformed into potent messages of presence by their communities, which in turn triggered spiritual and somatic effects in the pilgrims who journeyed to these newly sacralized locales.

EMMA ANDERSON

Foundational Events: Marian Apparitions and Their Aftermath

Healings at nineteenth-century Marian shrines were intimately related, both affectively and conceptually, to the events that had founded these places of pilgrimage. Indeed, Marian healings can be seen both as a ratification and as a reinterpretation of the Marian apparitions that preceded them. Marian apparitions are complex phenomena that are best thought of as a collective process of religious meaning-making that uses the ambiguous experiences of individuals as their foundation and inspiration. Nineteenth-century apparition sequences often began when young Catholics, usually of lowly origin, reported an encounter with an ambiguous figure variously described by them as a light, a cloud, a white object, or a female figure.[1] It is important to recognize that, in most cases, seers did not initially suggest that this figure was the Virgin Mary; rather, this identification often emerged as the result of a protracted period of negotiation between seers and their families, communities, and local church officials.[2] Sometimes this identification was accepted by the visionary only with

---

1. At Lourdes, Bernadette initially described the figure as "something white" that "had the shape of a little girl" (Sandra Zimdars-Swartz, *Encountering Mary: Visions of Mary from La Salette to Medjugorje* [New York: Avon, 1991], 47; Michael Carroll, *The Cult of the Virgin Mary: Psychological Origins* [Princeton: Princeton University Press, 1986], 156–58). At La Salette, the children reported seeing a white light, in which they gradually perceived the form of a woman weeping (Emma Anderson, "Changing Devotional Paradigms and Their Impact upon Nineteenth-Century Marian Apparitions: The Case of La Salette," *Union Seminary Quarterly Review* 52 [1998]: 108; Carroll, *Cult of the Virgin Mary*, 150; Zimdars-Swartz, *Encountering Mary*, 29). The children's description of this figure (particularly Melanie's) became progressively more detailed and emotional as time went on (Anderson, "Changing Devotional Paradigms," 118–19). Lucia's description of her apparition at Fatima similarly emphasized the figure's diminutive stature, luminosity, and unknown identity (Carroll, *Cult of the Virgin Mary*, 177–78).

2. At La Salette, it was the grandmother of the children's employer who first suggested that Melanie and Maximin had seen the Virgin Mary while they were taking care of cattle on the local mountainside, a suggestion that was seconded by the local parish priest (Michael Cox, *Rain for These Roots* [Milwaukee: Bruce, 1956], 4–5; Carroll, *Cult of the Virgin Mary*, 151). At Pontmain, it was the children's mother who initially suggested the identity of the apparition figure (Cheryl A. Porte, *Pontmain, Prophecy, and Protest: A Cultural-Historical Study of a Nineteenth-Century Apparition* [New York: Peter Lang, 2005], 2). At Lourdes, though it is not clear who first suggested the figure was the Virgin, it was not Bernadette, for, though she was repeatedly asked whether the figure was Mary, she continually replied that she did not know (Zimdars-Swartz, *Encountering Mary*, 49). Following these repeated suggestions, the figure's self-identification as "the Immaculate Conception" provided the confirmation many had sought. Similarly, Lucia, one of three young seers at Fatima, following her initial

---

considerable reluctance, if at all.[3] More than four years after his experiences, by which time the identification of his vision with the Virgin Mary was taken for granted by many Catholics, Maximin Giraud — one of the two young visionaries at La Salette — stated, "I do not know if it was the Blessed Virgin. I saw something . . . a lady."[4] Even Bernadette, that most iconic of nineteenth-century visionaries, initially responded to questions about the identity of the apparition figure by simply stating that she did not know, and she preferred throughout her life to call the figure she had seen Aquero (meaning simply "that one" or "her" in Bernadette's Bigourdan dialect). Moreover, she strongly resisted the artistic metastasization of the fourteen-year-old "little girl" she repeatedly encountered into more conventional, less personal devotional imagery of the Virgin Mary.[5]

But if young seers often did not initially interpret what they had experienced within a religious framework, then what are we to make of their experiences? Modern Marian apparitions have been interpreted by historians and social scientists as hallucinations of this-worldly female figures of personal import to

---

Marian apparition, stated, "I don't know if it was Our Lady. It was a very pretty little woman" (Carroll, *Cult of the Virgin Mary*, 177–78).

3. Michael Carroll, "The Virgin Mary at La Salette and Lourdes: Whom Did the Children See?" *Journal for the Scientific Study of Religion* 24 (1985): 56–73; Carroll, *Cult of the Virgin Mary*, 115–40; Anderson, "Changing Devotional Paradigms," 85–122; Zimdars-Swartz, *Encountering Mary*, 32.

4. J. Spencer Northcote, *Celebrated Sanctuaries of the Madonna* (Philadelphia: Peter F. Cunningham and Son, 1875), 236; Carroll, *Cult of the Virgin Mary*, 61; John S. Kennedy, "The Lady in Tears," in *A Woman Clothed with the Sun*, ed. John J. Delaney (Garden City, NY: Doubleday, 1961), 105. For a general discussion of seers' initial hypothesis about the identity of the apparition figure at La Salette, see Zimdars-Swartz, *Encountering Mary*, 29–32, and Anderson, "Changing Devotional Paradigms," 107–14.

5. Bernadette's refusal to identify the figure as the Virgin, and her dialect: Carroll, *Cult of the Virgin Mary*, 156–57; her description of the figure as a little girl and resistance to artistic reinterpretations of her vision: Ruth Harris, *Lourdes: Body and Spirit in the Secular Age* (London: Penguin, 1999), 57, 72–79; Carroll, *Cult of the Virgin Mary*, 157. For a thoughtful exploration of how contemporary female pilgrims to Fatima perceive and appropriate the Virgin Mary, in defiance of the Catholic Church's emphasis on her eternal virginity, see Lena Gemzöe, "The Feminization of Healing in Pilgrimage to Fátima," in *Pilgrimage and Healing*, ed. Jill Dubisch and Michael Winkelman (Tucson: University of Arizona Press, 2005). For popular appropriations of the figure of Mary Magdalene by New Age pilgrims to locales in southern France associated with her cult, see Anna Fedele, *Looking for Mary Magdalene: Alternative Pilgrimage and Ritual Creativity at Catholic Shrines in France* (New York: Oxford University Press, 2013). Such contemporary research reminds us that saintly figures are always in flux and that the meanings made of them can vary considerably from the approved interpretations of the church.

the individual seer.[6] Significantly, such experiences often seem to occur during a period of bereavement or separation from an important female figure in the seer's life. Stress, trauma, malnutrition, and illness have also been suggested as contributing factors to the raw experiences that became transformed by the seers' families and communities into theophanies in the hours, days, and weeks following the instigating events.[7] Gradually, seers' incoherent, vague, or ambiguous accounts of their experiences were unconsciously shaped both by their endless repetition and by the community's speculation and questioning into a coherent narrative, with a religious figure and message at its core. Though loosely based on the seers' original accounts, these reshaped accounts of what had occurred were strongly influenced by devotional imagery and the precedent of previous apparitions to lowly shepherd children.[8] Because they were a bricolage drawn from several sources, these crystallizing narratives often unselfconsciously contradicted, reinterpreted, or reshaped the children's original accounts to make them more coherent, compelling, and more obviously religious in tone.[9] Though they germinated from seers' experiences of personal trauma, loss, or deprivation, those apparition narratives that succeeded in at-

6. Carroll, *Cult of the Virgin Mary*, 117–29, 152–56, 157–64, 178–81; Porte, *Pontmain, Prophecy, and Protest*, 7–9; Anderson, "Changing Devotional Paradigms," 106–7.

7. For example, Carroll, *Cult of the Virgin Mary*, 152–53; Zimdars-Swartz, *Encountering Mary*, 31–32; and Anderson, "Changing Devotional Paradigms," 107–14, all suggest that the vision at La Salette, with its characteristic overtones of violence and deprivation, can be attributed to the domestic difficulties of its seers.

8. Carroll, *Cult of the Virgin Mary*, 134–36; Zimdars-Swartz, *Encountering Mary*, 38–39; David Blackbourn, *Marpingen: Apparitions of the Virgin Mary in a Nineteenth-Century German Village* (New York: Vintage, 1995). For a discussion of premodern Marian apparitions, see William Christian, *Apparitions in Late Medieval and Renaissance Spain* (Princeton: Princeton University Press, 1981).

9. During this process, anomalous elements were gradually challenged, excised, or reinterpreted. Maximin's original explanation of his vision at La Salette — that it involved an encounter with a woman weeping because she had been beaten by her son (William Ullathorne, *The Holy Mountain of La Salette* [Altamont, NY: La Salette, 1854], 44) — was collectively reinterpreted as meaning that Mary was actively restraining the chastising arm of her son, who wished to punish sinners. Moreover, the figure's harsh, even vindictive, tone was substantially softened in subsequent accounts to make it accord more closely with devotional expectations of Mary's behavior (Carroll, *Cult of the Virgin Mary*, 155–56; Anderson, "Changing Devotional Paradigms," 116–19). At Lourdes, the main point of controversy was Bernadette's insistence upon the diminutive stature and youth of the apparition figure, which Joseph Fabisch, in his creation of the iconic grotto statue that has come to be the definitive image of Lourdes, simply ignored (Harris, *Lourdes*, 72–74). For a thoughtful consideration of this process of collective negotiation of the themes, messages, and images of Marian apparitions, see Zimdars-Swartz, *Encountering Mary*, 11–16.

tracting a wide public following were ones that successfully recast idiosyncratic, personal contents into a clear, explicit message of powerful, sacred presence. The collective identification of the apparition figure as the Virgin Mary immediately reframed the sometimes bizarre accounts of visionaries into a miraculous breakthrough of the divine into the profane world that numinized its local point of entry.

It was this perception of Mary's continuing availability in the apparition locale, more than her reported words, that exerted a mesmerizing hold over the popular Catholic imagination and inspired the development of thaumaturgical cults at apparition sites: "The scenes of such manifestations are thought to be gaps in the curtain, tears in the veil, separating the two orders . . . the place of revelation continues to 'vibrate' with supernatural efficacy."[10] While the church hierarchy often focused upon the coherency and orthodoxy of the apparition's purported message, from the beginning, popular consensus held that apparitions were significant because they promised proximity to Mary's invisible yet tangible physical presence.[11] Whether at La Salette, Lourdes, or later, at Fatima, pilgrims flocked to be in the presence of the Mother of God and to imbibe the air, earth, and water that her advent had sacralized.[12] Though the preferred method of ingesting or physically immersing oneself in the sacred was through the medium of holy springs, which already had a strong association with otherworldly healing powers, a strong element of improvisation was also observable.[13] Having learned from Melanie and Maximin, the child visionaries at La Salette, that they had first seen the apparition figure seated, weeping, on a large rock, villagers began to chip off pieces of it to wear, ingest, sell, or soak

10. Victor Turner and Edith Turner, *Image and Pilgrimage in Christian Culture: Anthropological Perspectives* (New York: Columbia University Press, 1978), 206.

11. Ironically, even as pious crowds at apparition sites generally ignored theological niceties (except insofar as they confirmed the Virgin's identity), their perception of Mary's physical presence at apparition sites and their claims of its thaumaturgical effects helped set the stage for the official adoption of the Virgin's bodily assumption into heaven as the dogma of the church a century later, in 1950 (Barbara Corrado Pope, "Immaculate and Powerful: The Marian Revival in the Nineteenth Century," in *Immaculate and Powerful: The Female in Sacred Image and Social Reality*, ed. Clarissa Atkinson, Constance Buchanan, and Margaret Miles [Boston: Beacon, 1985], 190). Moreover, the visions of Catherine Labouré and Bernadette Soubirous were important in anticipating and confirming, respectively, the proclamation of the doctrine of the Immaculate Conception in 1854 (Thomas Kselman, *Miracles and Prophecies in Nineteenth-Century France* [New Brunswick, NJ: Rutgers University Press, 1983], 89–93).

12. Harris, *Lourdes*, 290–93.

13. Harris, *Lourdes*, 289–95; Pope, "Immaculate and Powerful," 180; Kselman, *Miracles and Prophecies*, 49; Zimdars-Swartz, *Encountering Mary*, 35–37.

in water, which they would then drink to obtain the corporeal and spiritual benefits of contact with the holy.[14] The alleged presence of the Virgin had made this stone into a contact relic as precious as the less accessible artifacts of her veil or belt, enshrined and unreachable in distant cathedrals.

If apparitions signaled, to the popular imagination, the earthly advent of the Mother of God, their serial, public nature in the nineteenth century further heightened the palpable sense of the Virgin's physical presence.[15] Whereas medieval and renaissance apparitions generally took place away from the public gaze, in the privacy of cloister, bedchamber, or pasture, in the nineteenth century apparitions became, for the first time, public, observable events.[16] At Lourdes (and later, at Fatima) hundreds of onlookers were present as the seer (or seers) saw and spoke with the apparition figure.[17] As the crowds were generally unable to perceive the apparition figure, the focus of their devotional attention shifted from Mary's invisible presence to the visible body of the seer in trance. Studying the demeanor, movements, and appearance of the visionary while in ecstasy became a way of perceiving, by proxy, the motions and intentions of the apparition figure, whom her seer was assumed to mirror or imitate. The faces of the seers in conversation with the Virgin were felt to take on the otherworldly beauty and luminosity of her own. Legions of the devout watched the expressions of the visionary and noted the direction and duration of her gaze for what it might reveal regarding the presence or behavior of her divine guest. Observation of the human side of such sacred encounters was pivotal in persuading many witnesses of the veracity of the seer's apparition experience and of the holy identity of the apparition figure.[18]

To their rapt observation of this dyadic interaction, many devotees added their own layer of interpretive imitation as they forged a cohesive set of behavioral prescriptions and ritual expectations at the apparition site. The assembled crowds at the apparition site often sought to share in the visionary's experience by mirroring the seer's reflective gestures: praying when she prayed, kneeling when she knelt, and standing when she stood. The crowd's

14. Zimdars-Swartz, *Encountering Mary*, 33–34. Similarly, at Fatima, leaves from the oak tree above which Mary allegedly appeared were taken as holy tokens by the crowd (Zimdars-Swartz, *Encountering Mary*, 80).

15. Zimdars-Swartz, *Encountering Mary*, 5–6.

16. Christian, *Apparitions*. Catherine Labouré's 1830 visions were more like these earlier, private revelations than the public, serial visions of Lourdes or Fatima (Zimdars-Swartz, *Encountering Mary*, 26–27).

17. Harris, *Lourdes*, 61–66.

18. Harris, *Lourdes*, 61–71; Zimdars-Swartz, *Encountering Mary*, 49–51.

imitative response to the seer's actions (which suggested a collective perception of the apparition figure that was not, in fact, the case) helped to foster a cohesive, prescriptive set of behaviors at a newly founded apparition site, which included maintaining silence, collectively praying the rosary, and carefully observing and imitating the seer's ritual gestures. These communal responses helped create an atmosphere that at once demonstrated and inculcated belief in the divine nature of the unfolding events.[19] Just as a seer's natal community often responded to their initial account by encouraging the religious elaboration of the emerging narrative, large crowds of the curious, by their devout demeanor at the apparition site, silently advocated for the credibility of the unfolding events, setting the stage for outbreaks of confirmatory, healing experiences.

Confirmatory Events:
Marian Healings as a Response to Perceived Presence

The ubiquitous emphasis upon healing at virtually all nineteenth-century Marian shrines is all the more striking because it was often not an explicit feature of apparition messages. Indeed, in some cases, such as La Salette, popular preoccupation with thaumaturgy existed in considerable tension with an apparition message that stressed punishment for unrepentant sinners rather than the miraculous release from physical suffering.[20] Exploitation of the thaumaturgical possibilities of the newly sacralized geography of apparition sites should thus be interpreted as a spontaneous, popular response to the Virgin's alleged physical presence. By drawing upon the ancient Catholic equation of immanence and miraculous power, devout crowds were to make healing phenomena the predominant preoccupation of many newly founded apparition shrines.

For invalids who either witnessed the ecstasies of Marian seers or visited, after the fact, sites that the Virgin's presence had hallowed, the Mother of God, always a part of their devotional life, seemed to become real to them or personally involved with them in a deeper and more primordial way. Catholic critics, stressing the universal nature of the church's message and the ubiquity of its sacramental system, objected that the ill encountered nothing at apparition locales

---

19. Kselman, *Miracles and Prophecies*, 145; Zimdars-Swartz, *Encountering Mary*, 50, 79. Moreover, rowdy or unruly crowds were punished by the apparition's failure to appear as promised (Harris, *Lourdes*, 66–67).

20. Anderson, "Changing Devotional Paradigms," 86, 99–100, 116; Zimdars-Swartz, *Encountering Mary*, 30–32; Kselman, *Miracles and Prophecies*, 62–68.

that they could not access through the devotional practices of their local parish. Invalids responded that on pilgrimage to sites where Mary had so recently manifested herself, they palpably felt her presence and were mysteriously drawn to a deepening of their spiritual relationship with her: "Sufferers recounted how they were remade, reborn, or resuscitated, how they were redefined by coming close to infinite power and grace. In essence, they described what twentieth-century philosophers would call an existential encounter with an infinite other."[21] Healings at Marian shrines in nineteenth-century Europe, whether they ameliorated physical, emotional, psychological, or relational ills, appear to have been precipitated by the individual invalid's cherished belief that the Mother of God could be physically encountered at the apparition site and that her "immaculate and powerful" presence had strong thaumaturgical implications.[22] Rituals of encounter with and in Mary's holy presence powerfully reshaped and reoriented the individual's whole self, "a totality of imagination, sensation, posture and bodily motion . . . through an existential process that depended entirely on a belief in the presence of the Virgin."[23] As invalids, in and through their bodies, mirrored seers' movements or drank or immersed themselves in waters sanctified by her theophany, many reported spiritual and physical effects upon their suffering bodies and minds.[24] These effects encompassed both physical healing, the amelioration or cessation of serious organic trauma or illness, and spiritual and relational healing, which, though it failed to alleviate physiological symptoms, gave the invalid and his or her family the grace to bear with increased tenacity, patience, and faith the realities of ongoing disability.[25]

Nineteenth-century Marian healings were thus profoundly relational events, deepening individual invalids' devotional engagement with the Virgin Mary even as they recast relations between *malades* and their families, often strained to the breaking point by years of suffering dependency. Illness, while in one sense a deeply individual crisis, also tests an invalid's relationship to his

21. Harris, *Lourdes*, 305.

22. My emphasis upon sufferers' perception of and response to holy presence as a critical factor in their experiences of physical, spiritual, and relational regeneration draws upon the work of a number of historians, anthropologists, and clinicians, including Robert Orsi, *Between Heaven and Earth: The Religious Worlds People Make and the Scholars Who Study Them* (Princeton: Princeton University Press, 2005); Orsi, *History and Presence* (Cambridge, MA: Harvard University Press, 2016); Thomas J. Csordas, *The Sacred Self: A Cultural Phenomenology of Charismatic Healing* (Berkeley: University of California Press, 1994); and James Dow, "Universal Aspects of Symbolic Healing: A Theoretical Synthesis," *American Anthropologist* 88 (1986): 56–66.

23. Harris, *Lourdes*, 311.

24. Kselman, *Miracles and Prophecies*, 46.

25. Pope, "Immaculate and Powerful," 192.

or her family members. As prolonged sickness or disability often brings with it the inability to work or share in the tasks of running a household, it entails, for the family, the double burden of caring for the invalid while simultaneously assuming his or her relinquished roles and duties. The stress of such a situation, difficult even in the short term, is almost unimaginably onerous when it becomes chronic. The relational toll exacted by illness suggests that, in addition to the actual symptoms of their physical condition, chronic invalids often suffer depression and guilt regarding their inability to function normally and express their perception that their continued dependency represents an unendurable burden for those closest to them. Family members of invalids, on the other hand, routinely express culpability for their impatience, lack of compassion, strong desire to abandon their responsibilities, and repulsion regarding the invalid's physical appearance or symptoms.[26]

Pilgrimage to and ritual engagement at Marian apparition sites directly addressed these familial strains by removing invalids and their family members from their routine roles and entrenched relational patterns and placing them in a liminal religious setting in which the *malade* was no longer secluded or socially marginal but ritually central. Their mutual endurance of the often grueling process of travel to these sites and their shared participation in cathartic rituals that actualized the living presence of the Virgin Mary often led invalids and those closest to them mutually to reaffirm their continuing value to one another, mitigating the invalid's profound sense of guilt and emotional and physical isolation.[27] Family members, for their part, drew strength from the sense that they were not alone in their difficult struggle to care for their ill or disabled family members, as Marian rituals both affirmed supernatural engagement and prompted a powerful sense of religiously inflected human solidarity or *communitas* with both the invalid and other families facing similar challenges.[28]

Marian healings, in their individual and collective dimensions, can be explored both as the logical consequence of Marian apparitions and as their inverse. As we have seen, Marian apparitions occurred when individual children's or adolescents' reports of unusual experiences and ambiguous phenomena were interpreted by their communities as a miraculous encounter with a sacred presence. The experiences of *miraculés* — or those invalids who experienced an amelioration of their physical, psychological, emotional, or relational traumas after

26. Kselman, *Miracles and Prophecies*, 40–43, 54–59.

27. Harris, *Lourdes*, 295; Turner and Turner, *Image and Pilgrimage*, 9–11.

28. Turner and Turner, *Image and Pilgrimage*, 250–51; Pope, "Immaculate and Powerful," 187–92; Kselman, *Miracles and Prophecies*, 44–47.

visiting Marian healing shrines — were predicated upon the experiences of these site-founding seers, as they had been collectively reinterpreted and propagated by seers' communities. Communal elaborations of Marian apparition narratives, despite their variety, uniformly emphasized the reality of Mary's enduring and puissant presence at her chosen apparition sites. It was invalids' strong belief that they stood in the presence of the thaumaturgical Mother of God, a belief predicated upon the emergent apparition narrative and confirmed by ritual gestures that emphasized thaumaturgical presence, which seems to have been most responsible for their experiences of physical, psychological, or relational healing. Moreover, both apparitions and healings took place in a public context in which the collective negotiation (in the case of Marian apparitions) or ratification (in the case of Marian healings) of their meaning was central to how both seers and invalids came to perceive and understand their own spiritual and somatic experiences.[29]

On the other hand, however, the experiences of seers and *miraculés* were the products of converse psychological processes of universalizing extrojection and personalizing introjection, respectively. The collective reinterpretation of seers' unusual experiences recast individual, idiosyncratic responses to trauma or loss into a clear narrative of religious encounter that had universal rather than merely personal significance. The healing experiences of *miraculés*, however, represented the converse process: individuals' encounter with a holy presence at Marian shrines could affect their physical, psychological, or spiritual well-being only when external, shared symbols, such as the Virgin herself, were introjected, making them personally and potently meaningful. The process of Marian healing thus involved a process of personal claiming or identification with public symbols, such that they became capable of touching and recasting an individual's most intimate spiritual, psychological, and physical realities. Though healings were similar to apparitions in their individual focus and psychological underpinnings, they thus involved contrasting psychological processes.

Occurring in the days, weeks, months, and years following the initiating apparition experiences, Marian healings were a solemn ratification of the spiritual validity of the controversial visionary experiences that had founded these new pilgrimage sites. Themselves seen as miraculous phenomena, they affirmed the divine identity of the apparition figure, cemented the developing apparition narrative, and represented a profound response to an environment that had been popularly redefined as sacred space.

29. Kselman, *Miracles and Prophecies*, 158.

The Interpretation of Marian Apparitions and Healings by the Church

The early elaboration of apparition narratives, the development of collective behavioral and ritual expectations at the apparition site, and the explosion of thaumaturgical outbreaks, which followed apparition events like aftershocks, took place in a setting where interpretive control of these events was still in the hands of seers and invalids, and also their families, communities, and local clergy. The upper echelons of the Catholic Church were initially absent from the interpretive fray due to their determination to maintain a discreet and cautious distance from unfolding events.[30] This caution, however, came at a price. When bishops did eventually step in to assert their episcopal authority and attempt to discern the nature and meaning of such incidents, they no longer encountered simply the original confused, ambiguous story of the young seers. Rather, tardy bishops confronted a coalescing apparition narrative centered upon a figure popularly perceived as being the Virgin Mary, an identification that seemed confirmed both by a devotional renaissance and by a rash of healings. Fueled by their belief in the palpable presence of the Mother of God among them, local communities had made of scanty, ambiguous evidence cults with fast-growing economic, social, and political roots in the local soil, and often in the national and international imagination.[31]

The often marked reluctance of the Catholic hierarchy to subject apparitions and healings to examination and analysis reflects the fact that the occurrence, scale, and increasingly public character of nineteenth-century Marian apparitions and healings presented them with a decidedly mixed blessing. On the one hand, apparitions and healings were perceived by some clerical observers as a literal godsend, as they often dramatically reversed plunging mass attendance and temporarily arrested the ongoing exodus of adult male parishioners. Impressed by the character and piety of seers and invalids, and by the pastoral effects of their experiences on the local parish, local clergy, relieved by their junior status of the need to make a definitive judgment upon their origin or nature, were free to enjoy the devotional renaissance that such incidents generally inspired. The successful popular transformation of ambiguous figures, messages, and corporeal manifestations into coherent, familiar religious images and rituals and the resultant rise in conventional devotional activity both helped incline

---

30. Pope, "Immaculate and Powerful," 178; Anderson, "Changing Devotional Paradigms," 90–91.

31. Harris, *Lourdes*, 84–91; Kselman, *Miracles and Prophecies*, 146–48; Zimdars-Swartz, *Encountering Mary*, 31–39; Nicholas Perry and Loreto Echeverría, *Under the Heel of Mary* (London: Routledge, 1988), 103.

local clergy, the church representatives closest to the community, toward belief in the divine origin of the events: "priests were influenced by the belief of their parishioners, and impressed by the pastoral effect of the new devotion."[32]

Moreover, apparitions and healings — which affirmed that miracles, through the holy agency of the Blessed Virgin, were possible even in the modern, secular age — were a profoundly attractive prospect to a church that increasingly sought to establish a defiantly antimodern, anti-ecumenical agenda that championed the prerogatives of Christ's mother, defended the possibility of modern miracles, and sought increasingly to defend the objective authority of the Papacy.[33] Promulgation of the doctrines of Mary's Immaculate Conception in 1854 (an event itself intimately related to the visionary activities of both Catherine Laboré and Bernadette Soubirous) and papal infallibility in 1870,[34] and the church's tardy placement of its imprimatur upon apparitions and healings across the continent, then, represented its conscious defiance of Protestantism, skepticism, and rationalism.[35]

As apparent as the phenomena's attractions, however, were their potential dangers. The bald fact that visions and healings were occurring without the sacramental intervention of the church presented an alarming prospect: that popular piety, rather than potentially reinvigorating Catholicism, was usurping for itself its sacred pantheon and prerogatives in its bypassing of traditional ritual venues and clerical authority.[36] If their potential benefits were to be reaped, such phenomena would have to be brought under the authority of the institutional church. The church's assertion of its exclusive right to judge the veracity of spiritual healings and of the unusual events that precipitated them was thus accompanied by its attempt to bring such phenomena under increased vigilance and place its own ritual stamp upon the proceedings at Marian healing venues, chiefly by making them more christocentric and sacramental. At Lourdes,

---

32. Kselman, *Miracles and Prophecies*, 143; see also 140–45. For the supportive reaction of local clergy at Lourdes, see Harris, *Lourdes*, 151–57; for La Salette, see Zimdars-Swartz, *Encountering Mary*, 37–39; Anderson, "Changing Devotional Paradigms," 89–91.

33. Pope, "Immaculate and Powerful," 182–83.

34. Carroll, *Cult of the Virgin Mary*, 162–64; Turner and Turner, *Image and Pilgrimage*, 227.

35. Pope, "Immaculate and Powerful," 175, 181–84; Porte, *Pontmain, Prophecy, and Protest*, xi; Victor Turner and Edith Turner, "Postindustrial Marian Pilgrimage," in *Mother Worship*, ed. James Preston (Chapel Hill: University of North Carolina Press, 1982), 152–53; Perry and Echeverría, *Under the Heel of Mary*, 115–18, 121–22; Anderson, "Changing Devotional Paradigms," 119.

36. Kselman, *Miracles and Prophecies*, 141, 159.

invalids' participation in the eucharistic parade gradually came to rival their immersion in its freezing waters as a ritual cue for the miraculous.[37]

Dangers arose not simply from the potential popular usurpation of clerical authority but by the high stakes involved in incorrect judgments in matters that had aroused considerable public attention. That the church might fail to recognize and celebrate a genuine manifestation of the divine was a serious possibility, as was the converse: that it might ratify what subsequent events would reveal to be a calculated fraud. Fears of the latter possibility were aroused when Maximin Giraud, the young seer at La Salette, began to market a liqueur he called "Salettine" after the church had already placed its imprimatur on his visions.[38]

Moreover, caution was natural given the fact that any episcopal ruling, no matter how circumspect, would be read in a polemical light by both devotional and skeptical audiences, each of whom the church wished, in some way, to court. It is immediately evident that the intensity of the collective interpretive process in the weeks following apparition and healing events, and the devotional fluorescence that they generated, created a strong popular expectation of episcopal ratification of the emergent cult. Popular lay opinion, irritated by the church's aloofness, would be inflamed by a negative decision, which might potentially alienate the church's base of support and risk the developing cult spiraling further away from clerical control.[39]

But why would the church be concerned about a possible positive decision enraging the very Protestant interlocutors and skeptical detractors whom its new dogmatic agenda seemed calculated to defy and irritate? Intriguingly, though Marian apparitions and healings were used to champion conservative theological developments, the form that this defense took increasingly utilized and backhandedly affirmed the medical and scientific views of the day, even when these standards ignored and contradicted the spiritual experiences of its own flock. Though the church enjoyed mocking the pretensions of medical science by contrasting its fallibility and impotence with the awesome healing powers of Christ and his mother, it nevertheless utilized, even privileged, in its own analysis of healing phenomena, many of the fledgling science's central assumptions and claims.

37. See Pope, "Immaculate and Powerful," 178; Kselman, *Miracles and Prophecies*, 48–49.

38. Turner and Turner, *Image and Pilgrimage*, 223; Perry and Echeverría; *Under the Heel of Mary*, 105. For a fascinating study of a fraudulent Marian apparition in nineteenth-century Germany, including its psychological and sociological dynamics, see Blackbourn, *Marpingen*.

39. Kselman, *Miracles and Prophecies*, 143–47, 153–55.

Contrasting Clerical and Popular Definitions of Miraculous Healing

While initially aloof from the healing furor, eventually the hierarchy stepped in to rule on both the instigatory apparitions and the rash of somatic and spiritual responses they had engendered. At first, episcopal committees were largely guided by Benedict XIV's Enlightenment-influenced writings on miracles, which had been formulated to adjudicate the evaluation of potential saints and stated that, to be considered miraculous, a healing must have resisted conventional cures, and that the miraculous cure itself should be instantaneous, otherwise inexplicable, and "perfect" or total.[40] As the nineteenth century progressed, this already somatically focused, rigid standard would become even more exacting as it was more and more influenced by "the need for scientific verification and . . . many of the epistemological criteria of modern medicine."[41] Beginning in the 1870s, clerical examiners began to request that sick pilgrims to Lourdes who wished to have their experiences officially recognized as miracles bring with them a certificate from a competent medical authority describing their complaint, the range of treatment options utilized, and the degree of success attained. In effect, participating doctors were required to confess in writing their inability substantially to ameliorate their patient's medical condition, thus giving the medical profession an important role in "testifying to its own helplessness."[42] After their allegedly miraculous encounter, patients were reexamined by medical authorities to ensure that the physiological results they claimed to have experienced were valid, apparently permanent, and medically inexplicable.[43]

These de facto definitions of miraculous healing adopted by the Catholic hierarchy are as interesting for what they encompass as for what they exclude. By requiring the participation of the medical establishment to certify the incurable nature of the invalid's complaint, and their acknowledgment of the reality of its amelioration and its medical inexplicability, the church was attempting to force medical elites both to acknowledge the limits of their own capabilities and to recognize the reality of supernatural intervention in certain cases. In effect, the Catholic hierarchy was attempting to utilize the status and perceived objectivity of medical professionals to persuade the undecided about the possibility of miracles in the modern age. The church engaged with biomedicine

40. Harris, *Lourdes*, 321–22.

41. Harris, *Lourdes*, 307.

42. Kselman, *Miracles and Prophecies*, 41–43.

43. Harris, *Lourdes*, 307. For more on the gradual shift from clerical to medical judgment of Marian cures, see Harris, *Lourdes*, 293–304; Kselman, *Miracles and Prophecies*, 41–42.

because it wished to present Marian healings as "empirically verifiable events" or "facts,"[44] which could be objectively proven through rigorous standards of evaluation and analysis, thus earning the hard-won credulity of those beyond the devotional boundaries of Catholicism.

Equally evident, however, is what was sacrificed in the hierarchy's quest for scientific legitimacy in their investigation of Marian cures. The restriction of the discussion of "the miraculous" solely to cases in which there had been an inexplicable, sudden, somatic amelioration of serious illness or injury in the face of medical impotence had several important implications. First, such a construction of the relationship between the medical and the spiritual seemed to posit that they could never work together. By requiring that doctors admit that, in their opinion, an individual's cure was impossible, Catholicism took upon itself the role of one of its principal saints, Saint Jude, assuming patronage only of those who had no hope for the medical amelioration of their symptoms and had become lost causes. Such a restriction implied that the many cases of illness or injury that responded to the pedestrian overtures of conventional medicine were devoid of any supernatural component. In seeking medical confirmation of its supernatural agenda, the hierarchy had inadvertently restricted the role of the divine.

Second, by making medical testimony critical to the judgment of miraculous experiences at Marian shrines, the late nineteenth-century church displayed either its ignorance of or its lack of appreciation for the seriousness of the economic and geographic barriers facing much of their rural flock in their increasing frustrating search for competent medical care. Health care, particularly in remote rural locations, was often either nonexistent or so exorbitant that it was out of reach of the majority.[45] Many rural poor frequented Marian shrines, local curés, or reputedly healing waters because they lacked the financial means to consult expensive medical practitioners, who were becoming increasingly rare in rural areas over the course of the nineteenth century.[46] Moreover, some rural Catholics who enjoyed both access to doctors and the ability to pay for their often dubious expertise chose instead to visit Catholic shrines because they believed (apparently unlike the Catholic hierarchy) in the supernatural etiology

---

44. Kselman, *Miracles and Prophecies*, 160; Pope, "Immaculate and Powerful," 190.

45. Kselman, *Miracles and Prophecies*, 37–39; Harris, *Lourdes*, 290–94.

46. According to Kselman, *Miracles and Prophecies*, 38, the number of doctors in France declined in the second half of the nineteenth century, from 18,099 in 1847 to 14,538 in 1896. For the inadequacies of biomedicine in nineteenth-century France, see Kselman, *Miracles and Prophecies*, 37–40; Harris, *Lourdes*, 294–95.

of their illness and thus, quite logically, in the possibility of its supernatural amelioration.[47]

Third, and most profoundly, the Catholic hierarchy's conversation with biomedicine, by restricting consideration of the miraculous solely to its measurable, somatic elements, removed Marian healing from the wider penumbra of spiritual and relational associations it had come to acquire in the popular context. Its attempts to force its critics to recognize the impartiality of its evaluative methods led the hierarchy effectively to ignore the often profound spiritual experiences of their own congregants (though this decision was reciprocal: as many of those who experienced what they considered to be miraculous interventions refused to submit themselves to the onerous process of clerical questioning and medical verification).[48] As we have seen, popular nineteenth-century perceptions of Marian healing, though they centered upon the corporeal (Mary's invisible yet palpable physical presence, the bodily movements of the seer, the answering somatic motions of the crowd, and the hope for the physical amelioration of illness), were nonetheless broad and generous in their definition. Healing, in the understanding of lay Catholics, encompassed *both* the miraculous cessation of physical suffering *and* an invalid's renewed sense of personal and relational strength, inspired by a deepening of their relationship to the Virgin and a renewal of their affective ties to their families and communities. In the absence of a dramatic, medically inexplicable cessation of their physical symptoms, many credited their pilgrimage with precipitating important changes in the way that they and their families were able to meet the ongoing challenge of illness and suffering. The hierarchy, due to their rigid, stringent definition of the miraculous, was unable to address these more diffuse, yet equally profound experiences of healing. In attempting to shape a definition of the miraculous that would contrast divine intervention with medical impotence, the upper rungs of the church turned their collective back on the experiences of the vast majority of Catholic pilgrims: "both medical and clerical authorities sought to limit too closely the experience of cure, placing 'objective' criteria on a polymorphous and often intensely subjective experience that was best validated, not by 'experts' but rather by individuals, their families and communities."[49]

<hr/>

47. Kselman, *Miracles and Prophecies*, 39–40; Harris, *Lourdes*, 290–93.

48. Harris, *Lourdes*, 307. Gemzöe's research ("Feminization of Healing") on popular perception of healing at today's Fatima shrine hints at a similar contemporary divide.

49. Harris, *Lourdes*, 289.

Conclusion

The Marian cures that unfolded at nineteenth-century apparition sites involved the perception of holy presence and the affirmation and deepening of existing relationships "between heaven and earth" and within families.[50] Marian healings were a somatic, spiritual, and relational expression of an ongoing communal process of interpretation that sought to make comprehensible and universally meaningful the anomalous experiences of children and young people who had disclosed their ambiguous encounter with a form, a light, or a "lady." The community recast visionaries' experiences as theophanic manifestations in which Mary's ongoing physical presence was seen as impregnating with holy power the air, earth, and water of the apparition site. As well as recasting their experiences in theological terms, seers' communities often reflected or mirrored visionaries' physical postures and gestures during serial apparition sequences to create both an atmosphere of belief and a strong sense of collective perception of and response to the apparition figure. In healings, this perception of presence was even more powerfully expressed. An individual invalid's encounter with Mary at her newly founded shrine facilitated his or her personalization of shared religious symbols such that they became "transactional" — able to affect his or her psychological, physiological, and spiritual realities.[51] But such cures were also cathartic "social dramas,"[52] in which the profound alienation experienced by many invalids — and the painfully ambivalent emotions of pity, guilt, anger, and fear that their suffering dependency provoked in their families and communities — could be transformed through the collective experiences of shared ritual into a powerful new sense of social solidarity or *communitas*.[53] Enacted in a liminal context that challenged entrenched devotional, familial, and social dynamics, rituals that evoked and celebrated the active, healing presence of the Virgin Mary could palpably affect an individual invalid's somatic condition and familial relationships.

While lay Catholic communities forged cohesive religious narratives from the raw material of seers' fragmentary accounts and imposed upon crowds of the curious informal ritual practices that instilled and celebrated a sense of thaumaturgical presence, the Catholic hierarchy sought to utilize apparitions

---

50. Orsi, *Between Heaven and Earth*.

51. Dow, "Universal Aspects of Symbolic Healing," 60.

52. Kselman, *Miracles and Prophecies*, 37–40; Pope, "Immaculate and Powerful," 178.

53. Turner and Turner, *Image and Pilgrimage*, 250–52; Kselman, *Miracles and Prophecies*, 37–46; Pope, "Immaculate and Powerful," 187–92.

and healings in their defensive dialogue with modernity. In its investigation of the purportedly miraculous healings at Marian shrines, the Catholic Church utilized a narrow, somatic definition of the miraculous that made it possible for them to demand that the medical establishment acknowledge the limits of its ability and recognize the reality of supernatural intervention. But this exclusively physical definition of Marian miracles, while allowing dialogue with the medical community, simultaneously hampered the hierarchy's ability to comprehend or accept their flock's more diffuse, holistic definitions and experiences of Marian healings.

3

Healing, Belief, and Interpretation in Nineteenth-Century Protestant America

Heather D. Curtis

S piritual healing was the subject of intense debate among late nineteenth-century Protestants, and, as this chapter will reveal, the contrasts and commonalities with events in Catholic Europe are particularly instructive for contemporary debates about the hermeneutics of healing. During this period, several competing movements devoted to the promotion and practice of divine or metaphysical healing emerged and spread rapidly across North America, Great Britain, and Europe. Members of the scientific community who were attempting to bolster and solidify their authority over the process of diagnosing and treating sickness in these same years often responded to proponents of spiritual healing with skepticism and hostility. Within this context, contests over the proper interpretations of illness, health, and healing proliferated.[1]

The author gratefully acknowledges support for this essay from a John Templeton Foundation Postdoctoral Fellowship and a Summer Research Fellowship from the Mary Baker Eddy Library for the Betterment of Humanity, Boston, MA.

1. Throughout this essay, *spiritual healing* is used in a manner consistent with the definition put forward by Sarah Coakley in her introduction to this volume: movements and claims of spiritual healing in nineteenth-century North America and Great Britain involved experiences of healing directly attributed to God. Both divine- and metaphysical-healing movements fall within this definitional rubric. *Healing*, as Coakley suggests in her opening reflections, is a multivalent term that is often the subject of definitional disagreement. One of the main goals of this essay is to parse debates about the meaning of healing in the late nineteenth century, particularly between scientists who attempted to identify healing with curing (the elimination of physiological disease), on the one hand, and proponents of spiritual healing, who advocated a more elastic or comprehensive definition, on the other.

This essay explores how participants in faith cure and Christian Science — two of the most prominent spiritual healing movements to arise during the latter decades of the nineteenth century — defined, discerned, and defended the meaning and experience of healing within the increasingly scientific and skeptical cultural milieu of late nineteenth-century North America and Great Britain.[2] Highlighting the intriguing and often-overlooked similarities between Christian Science and faith cure, while at the same time noting the important distinctions in their theories and practices of healing, demonstrates that the fluid and unhierarchical structure of late nineteenth-century American and British Protestantism, as opposed to that of Roman Catholicism, allowed for creativity and contestation in the process of interpreting spiritual healing. Although leaders of these rival movements disagreed about the nature of embodied reality and, consequently, about the precise theological meaning of miraculous healing, they shared a conviction that instances of physical restoration provided a powerful antidote to scientific naturalism, materialism, and agnosticism.

Examining how proponents of divine healing and Christian Science sought to counter the swelling unbelief of the modern era through their theories and practices of healing reveals a curious paradox in their attitudes toward scientific empiricism. Even as they insisted that experiences of bodily recovery supplied proof of prayer's efficacy and confirmation of God's presence and power in the modern period, they simultaneously questioned the sufficiency of empirical evidence for ascertaining spiritual realities. Healing, according to these late nineteenth-century Protestants, encompassed much more than somatic improvement. Restoring the body to health required reorienting the mind and reforming the soul. To focus on observable signs of corporeal remediation as the chief measure of God's activity in response to prayer, therefore, was to overlook the mental and spiritual transformations that healing entailed. In order to grasp the broader meaning and implications of either Christian Science or faith cure, leaders of these movements asserted, sufferers seeking healing had to develop spiritual discernment through the disciplined practice of prayer. Only when they embraced a hermeneutics of healing that valued the spiritual over the material,

---

2. While some historians have argued that *faith cure* was a derogative label applied to the movement only by critics, I find evidence of its use among participants, especially during the first two decades of the movement's history. As the movement came under increasing attack in the mid- to late 1880s, some of its defenders began to distance themselves from the phrase *faith cure* and argued that *divine healing* represented a more appropriate moniker. Given the enduring popularity of *faith cure* among many participants throughout the 1880s, I have chosen to use *divine healing* and *faith cure* interchangeably.

the metaphysical over the natural, and the ineffable over the empirical would ailing individuals truly experience divine healing for body, mind, and soul.

Proving the Power of Prayer: Healing as Empirical Evidence of God's Presence and Potency

In the summer of 1872, the eminent British physicist John Tyndall proposed "an experimental test" to ascertain "the value of prayer on behalf of the sick."[3] Tyndall issued his proposition amidst growing interest in spiritual healing among European, British, and North American Protestants.[4] While accounts of miraculous cure had always been part of the Christian tradition, until the mid-nineteenth century, many Protestants viewed these events as exceptional, believing that the age of miracles had ceased at the conclusion of the biblical era and assuming, therefore, that God healed primarily through natural means rather than supernatural intervention. Beginning in the 1850s and 60s, however, reports of "marvelous cures" taking place at various locations in Europe began to circulate with increasing frequency throughout Great Britain and the United States, prompting a number of Protestant clergy and lay people to reassess God's willingness and ability to perform miracles of healing in the modern period.[5] By December of 1871, when the Prince of Wales recovered from a severe bout of cholera after special petitions for his healing were offered in churches throughout the realm, believers on both sides of the Atlantic boldly credited his restoration to direct, divine intervention in response to intercessory prayer.[6]

---

3. "The 'Prayer for the Sick.' Hints Toward a Serious Attempt to Estimate its Value," in *The Prayer Gauge Debate by Prof. Tyndall, Francis Galton, and Others . . .* , ed. John O. Means (Boston: Congregational Publishing Society, 1876), 9–19; originally published in *The (London) Contemporary Review* (July 1872): 205–10; and "By the Author of 'Hints Toward a Serious Attempt to Estimate the Value of the "Prayer for the Sick,"'" in *The Prayer Gauge Debate by Prof. Tyndall, Francis Galton, and Others . . .* , ed. Means, 116–35; originally published in *The (London) Contemporary Review* (October 1872).

4. Proponents of divine and metaphysical healing identified God as the source of healing and fall within the rubric of spiritual healing as defined in this volume.

5. For an overview of Protestant beliefs regarding the miraculous in the nineteenth century, see Robert Bruce Mullin, *Miracles and the Modern Religious Imagination* (New Haven: Yale University Press, 1996), esp. 9–30. On the circulation of healing testimonies in mid-nineteenth-century Britain, see *Dorothea Trudel, or, The Prayer of Faith. With Some Particulars of the Remarkable Manner in Which Large Numbers of Sick Persons Were Healed in Answer to Special Prayer* (London: Morgan and Chase, n.d.), 1.

6. On the illness and recovery of the Prince of Wales, see Robert Bruce Mullin, "Science,

As a prominent member of the British scientific community and a thoroughgoing naturalist, Tyndall doubted that the outpouring of prayer on Edward's behalf had anything to do with the prince's recovery. Skeptical about all explanations of physical healing that involved abrogation of the natural order, Tyndall insisted that claims about the "intrusion of supernatural power in answer to the petitions of men" be subjected to rigorous empirical analysis and verified in "tangible form." In an article entitled "The 'Prayer for the Sick.' Hints Toward a Serious Attempt to Estimate its Value," published in the July 1872 edition of London's *Contemporary Review*, Tyndall suggested that a hospital ward housing patients afflicted with "those diseases which have been best studied, and of which the mortality-rates are best known" be "made the object of special prayer by the whole body of the faithful" for a period of three to five years, during which time the patients would also receive "the care of first-rate physicians." "At the end of that time, the mortality-rates should be compared with the past rates, and also with that of other leading hospitals similarly well managed during the same period." Such a study, Tyndall contended, would allow investigators to ascertain the "calculable value of prayer" through "clinical observation," enabling them to "estimate" and "measure" the power of intercession to produce "physical results."[7]

Tyndall's proposal ignited a vigorous transatlantic controversy over the role of prayer and divine intervention in the healing process. Scientists, clergymen, and laypersons debated whether "the efficacy of prayer" represented a "legitimate subject of scientific inquiry," queried the ethical implications of conducting an experiment that encouraged prayer for only a select group of individuals, and argued over the question whether empirical changes in physical condition constituted necessary or valid "evidence" of God's supernatural activity. Some critics accused Tyndall of arrogance and blasphemy, arguing that the notion of putting God to the test was not only inappropriate but also irreverent. Indeed, over the next decade, Protestant believers in both Britain and North America

---

Miracles and the Prayer Gauge Debate," in *When Science and Christianity Meet*, ed. David C. Lindberg and Ronald L. Numbers (Chicago: University of Chicago Press, 2003), 203–24; and Rick Ostrander, *The Life of Prayer in a World of Science: Protestants, Prayer, and American Culture, 1870–1930* (New York: Oxford University Press, 2000), 18–19.

7. "The 'Prayer for the Sick. Hints Toward a Serious Attempt to Estimate its Value," 9–19. Although this paper appeared anonymously in London's *Contemporary Review*, authorship was generally attributed to Sir Henry Thompson, a renowned surgeon and professor of medicine. Tyndall wrote a preface for the article and subsequently received credit for originating and promoting the proposal.

increasingly associated Tyndall's name with religious skepticism, scientific naturalism, and materialistic philosophy.[8]

While resistance to the idea of conducting a "prayer-gauge" experiment remained strong among many Protestants for both theological and ethical reasons, Tyndall's proposal also provoked widespread and determined efforts to demonstrate that God did, in fact, heal in response to intercessory petition. In the years immediately following the publication of Tyndall's challenge, testimonies of God's ongoing, tangible, and often miraculous answers to prayer for bodily restoration poured into popular religious periodicals and newspapers. Protestant leaders such as William Patton — a widely respected Congregationalist minister, editor, and Howard University president — compiled lengthy anthologies containing hundreds of answered-prayer narratives, including numerous accounts of physical cure.[9]

The notion that experiences of healing proved God's presence and power to heal in the modern era was a central theme in the discourse of both Christian Science and divine healing as they emerged and developed over the course of the 1870s and 80s.[10] Although leaders of these competing movements consistently

---

8. Francis Galton, "Statistical Inquiries into the Efficacy of Prayer," in *The Prayer Gauge Debate by Prof. Tyndall, Francis Galton, and Others...*, ed. Means, 85–106. For overviews of this controversy, see Mullin, *Miracles*, 45–46; Mullin, "Science, Miracles, and the Prayer-Gauge Debate," esp. 210–21; and Ostrander, *Life of Prayer*, ch. 1.

9. William W. Patton, *Prayer and Its Remarkable Answers: Being a Statement of Facts in the Light of Reason and Revelation* (New York: Funk and Wagnalls, 1885). For a discussion of "answered prayer narratives" as a response to Tyndall's proposal, see Mullin, "Science, Miracles, and the Prayer-Gauge Debate," 219–21; and Ostrander, *Life of Prayer*, ch. 1.

10. For historical accounts of the birth and growth of Christian Science, see Stephen Gottschalk, *The Emergence of Christian Science in American Religious Life* (Berkeley: University of California Press, 1973); Gillian Gill, *Mary Baker Eddy* (Reading, MA: Perseus, 1998); and Robert Peel, *Mary Baker Eddy*, 3 vols. (New York: Holt, Rinehart and Winston, 1972–80, c. 1966–77). Recent histories of the divine healing movement include Jonathan R. Baer, "Perfectly Empowered Bodies: Divine Healing in Modernizing America" (PhD diss., Yale University, 2002); Paul G. Chappell, "The Divine Healing Movement in America" (PhD diss., Drew University, 1983); Heather D. Curtis, *Faith in the Great Physician: Suffering and Divine Healing in American Culture, 1860–1900* (Baltimore: Johns Hopkins University Press, 2007); Nancy Hardesty, *Faith Cure: Divine Healing in the Holiness and Pentecostal Movements* (Peabody, MA: Hendrickson, 2003); James W. Opp, *The Lord for the Body: Religion, Medicine, and Protestant Faith Healing in Canada, 1880–1930* (Montreal: McGill-Queen's University Press, 2005); and James Robinson, *Divine Healing: The Formative Years, 1830–1880; Theological Roots in the Transatlantic World* (Eugene, OR: Wipf & Stock, 2011) and *Divine Healing: The Holiness-Pentecostal Transition Years, 1890–1906; Theological Transposition in the Transatlantic World* (Eugene, OR: Wipf & Stock, 2013).

and often virulently stressed their sharp theological and practical differences, many of their contemporaries — critics and supporters alike — highlighted the apparent commonalities. Chief among these similarities was the stance that exponents of divine healing and Christian Science adopted toward scientific naturalism. "'Faith cure' and 'mind cure' and 'Christian Science,'" Congregationalist minister Lyman Abbott remarked, "are natural, and in the main healthful, reactions against materialism." Although they usually bristled when commentators lumped their movements together, advocates of faith cure and Christian Science would have been hard pressed to dispute Abbott's observation.[11]

From the beginning, Mary Baker Eddy (1821–1910) conceived of Christian Science as a refutation of materialistic science, philosophy, and religion. Although she dated her discovery of "the Science of divine metaphysical healing" to 1866, she spent several years working out the implications of her insights before beginning to teach and proclaim the theory and practice that she eventually named "Christian Science." She accepted her first students in 1870 and published the first edition of *Science and Health*, the textbook that laid out the principles of her "metaphysics," in 1875. Eddy and a small group of followers founded the first Church of Christ, Scientist, in Boston in 1879. Two years later, the Massachusetts Metaphysical College opened its doors to students seeking training in the teaching and methods of Christian Science healing. In 1883, Eddy established the monthly *Journal of Christian Science*, which included articles explaining the principles of mind cure alongside numerous testimonies of physical healing. Over the next fifteen years, Christian Science expanded outward from its epicenter in Boston as practitioners organized institutes of healing and formal associations for spreading Eddy's teachings throughout the United States and Canada.[12]

Eddy's earliest writings on her theory of healing reveal that she regarded Tyndall as the primary spokesperson for modern materialism and her principal adversary. "New positions of thought have already gained a hearing," Eddy maintained in *Moral Science*, a document she used as the basis for her teaching in the early 1870s. "One is that all is matter; the other that all is mind. Prof. Tyndall entertains the first, I the last; let us then according to the saying of the great general, 'fight it out on this line.'"[13] In the introduction to the first revised edition of *Science and Health*, published in 1878, Eddy again invoked Tyndall's

11. Lyman Abbott, as quoted in *Christian Science Journal* 10, no. 9 (December 1892): 413.

12. This history is recounted in various places, including Gottschalk, *Emergence of Christian Science*; Gill, *Mary Baker Eddy*; and Peel, *Mary Baker Eddy*.

13. Mary Baker Glover, *Moral Science*, 35, Articles and Manuscripts Collection, Accession:A11396, Mary Baker Eddy Library for the Betterment of Humanity, Boston, MA.

name, alongside those of "Huxley, Darwin, and all the honored array of materialistic philosophers," who "have thrown the glove, and challenged to combat physics and Metaphysics."[14]

Healing, Eddy claimed, was the most effective weapon that she wielded in the battle to demonstrate the superiority of Christian Science over scientific materialism. "Several years ago we made the Metaphysical discovery that mind governs the body not in part, but the whole, and submitted our radical statement of this to the severest practical tests. Since which our theory has gradually gained ground, and become known as the most effectual curative agent," she wrote. Instances of healing through the practice of Christian Science, Eddy contended, offered empirical confirmation that her "Metaphysical method of cure" trumped all forms of medical and philosophical materialism. "Nothing in pathology has gone beyond the results that we have effected through mind alone in changing the secretions of the system, renewing the structure, and preventing as well as curing disease . . . ," she declared, "giving proof to this world, in evidence indisputable, that Metaphysics walks over physics in healing the sick, and bringing out the latent possibilities of our being."[15]

Although Eddy and her disciples dismissed Tyndall's sort of "prayer-gauge tests" as "unchristian" and worthy of "vehement rebuke," they simultaneously insisted that cases of cures wrought through Christian Science demonstrated the truth of "divine power" over the illusion of material reality in the modern era.[16] The purpose of Christian Science, Eddy and her followers argued, was "to reinstate primitive Christianity and its lost element of healing." By reviving the healing theory and practices of Jesus and the apostles, Christian Scientists provided "proof that Christian promises were to be fulfilled in the present," as historian Stephen Gottschalk has put it, and gave participants "a sense of the immediacy of divine power."[17] To this end, Eddy encouraged practitioners and beneficiaries of her metaphysical Science to bear witness to their experiences of physical restoration. "Testimony in regard to healing of the sick is highly important," she stated in the manual for the Church of Christ, Scientist. "More than a mere rehearsal of blessings, it scales the pinnacles of praise and illustrates the demonstration of Christ."[18]

---

14. Mary Baker Eddy, *Science and Health* (Lynn, MA: Dr. Asa G. Eddy, 1878), 2:2–3.

15. Eddy, *Science and Health*, 2:2–4.

16. "Faith Work, Christian Science, and Other Cures," *Christian Science Journal* 3, no. 5 (August 1885): 91.

17. On Christian Science healing as a primitivist impulse, see Gottschalk, *Emergence of Christian Science*, esp. 23–24, 210–11, 237–38.

18. Quoted in Gottschalk, *Emergence of Christian Science*, 221.

For Eddy and her followers, experiences of bodily cure confirmed that a "practical, spiritual Christianity, with its healing power" would triumph over the "modern materialistic" philosophy of naturalists like Tyndall by beating them at their own game. Empirical evidence of "the supremacy of Spirit" over matter, of God's willingness and ability to restore ailing bodies to health abounded, Eddy asserted. "Once seen," she argued, this "proof" led to the incontrovertible conclusion that "Mind is All-in-all, that the only realities are the divine Mind and idea," that the "materialistic view" was an "error, consisting chiefly of sin, sickness and death, that must yield to harmony and Life at last."[19]

In contrast to Christian Science, faith cure had no single founder or primary leader. The practice of divine healing initially emerged in the 1850s among European Pietists who encouraged sick persons to put their faith in God as the "great physician" who promised both spiritual and physical redemption to believers in scriptural passages such as Exodus 15:26, "I am the LORD that healeth thee," and James 5:15, "the prayer of faith shall save the sick, and the Lord shall raise him up" (King James Version). During the 1860s, news of the "remarkable manner in which large numbers of sick persons were healed in answer to prayer" at Mannedorf, Switzerland, and at several locales in Germany spread to British and American Protestants. By 1875, leaders from a number of Protestant denominations had embraced divine healing.[20]

Converts to faith cure included prominent figures such as Episcopal layman Charles Cullis (1833–92), a homeopathic physician who founded and directed a network of health, welfare, and healing institutions in Boston; the Reverend John Inskip (1816–84), Methodist leader and president of the National Camp Meeting Association for the Promotion of Holiness; Presbyterian minister William E. Boardman (1810–96), author of the popular tract *The Higher Christian Life*; the Reverend A. J. Gordon (1836–95), pastor of Boston's Clarendon Street Baptist Church and an important participant in late nineteenth-century evangelical

19. Mary Baker Eddy, *Christian Science: No and Yes*, 8th rev. ed. (Boston: W. G. Nixon, 1891), 46; Mary Baker Eddy, "Metaphysical Science," *Ipswich Chronicle* (c. 1877), Scrapbook 1A, Mary Baker Eddy Scrapbooks Collection, Mary Baker Eddy Library for the Betterment of Humanity, Boston, MA; Mary Baker Eddy, *Science and Health*, 3rd rev. ed. (Lynn, MA: Dr. Asa G. Eddy, 1881), 9; Mary Baker Eddy, *Science and Health with Key to the Scriptures* (Boston: The Mary Baker Eddy Foundation, 1910), 109; and Glover, *Moral Science*, 35.

20. For a contemporary account of how news of divine healing spread during this period, see Charles Cullis, introduction to *Dorothea Trudel; or, The Prayer of Faith*, rev. ed. (Boston: Willard Tract Repository, 1872). Fuller histories of the movement's development may be found in Baer, "Perfectly Empowered Bodies"; Chappell, "Divine Healing Movement in America"; Curtis, *Faith in the Great Physician*; Hardesty, *Faith Cure*; Opp, *Lord for the Body*; and Robinson, *Divine Healing*.

movements such as temperance, foreign missions, and D. L. Moody's revivals; and A. B. Simpson (1843–1919), a Presbyterian minister who would eventually become the minister of the nondenominational Gospel Tabernacle church in New York City and the founder of the Christian and Missionary Alliance.[21]

While many apologists for faith healing were male ministers, women played vital roles in shaping the movement's theology and practice. Women who served in important leadership positions included Episcopalian Carrie Judd Montgomery (1858–1946), author of one of the pivotal texts on divine healing and editor of a popular periodical promoting healing and holiness; Mary Mossman (c. 1826–after 1909), who established and operated a healing home at the popular holiness seaside retreat in Ocean Grove, New Jersey; Elizabeth Baxter (1837–1926), author, preacher, and cofounder of the Bethshan house of healing in London, England; S. L. Lindenberger, "house mother" of a large faith home in New York City; and Sarah Mix (1832–84), an African American Adventist who ministered to the sick throughout New England.[22]

During the 1880s, the divine healing movement grew rapidly as proponents conducted healing services at camp meetings and faith conventions, founded numerous faith homes for invalids who desired to seek healing in a nurturing environment, published treatises defending faith cure theology, and launched

---

21. For fuller biographical treatments of these figures and discussions of their participation in divine healing, see Curtis, *Faith in the Great Physician*; William E. Boardman, *Faith-Work under Dr. Cullis, in Boston* (Boston: Willard Tract Repository, 1874); W. H. Daniels, ed., *Dr. Cullis and His Work: Twenty Years of Blessing in Answer to Prayer* (1885; repr., New York: Garland, 1985); William McDonald, *The Life of Rev. John S. Inskip* (1885; repr., New York: Garland, 1985); Mrs. [Mary M. Adams] Boardman, *Life and Labours of the Rev. W. E. Boardman* (New York: D. Appleton, 1887); Adoniram Judson Gordon, *The Ministry of Healing: or, Miracles of Cure for All Ages* (Boston: Howard Gannett, 1882); Ernest B. Gordon, *Adoniram Judson Gordon: A Biography* (New York: Fleming H. Revell, 1896); A. B. Simpson, *The Gospel of Healing*, rev. ed. (1888; repr., London: Morgan and Scott, 1915); and A. E. Thompson, *The Life of A. B. Simpson: Official Authorized Edition* (New York: Christian Alliance, 1920).

22. Like their male counterparts, many female leaders also authored accounts of their own experiences, and some inspired biographies. See, for example, Carrie F. Judd, *The Prayer of Faith* (1880; repr. in *The Life and Teachings of Carrie Judd Montgomery* [New York: Garland, 1985]); Carrie Judd Montgomery, *Under His Wings: The Story of My Life* (1936; repr. in *The Life and Teachings of Carrie Judd Montgomery*); Mary H. Mossman, *Steppings in God; or, The Hidden Life Made Manifest* (New York: Eaton and Mains, 1909); Nathaniel Wiseman, *Elizabeth Baxter (Wife of Michael Paget Baxter), Saint, Evangelist, Preacher, Teacher, and Expositor* (London: Christian Herald, 1928); S. A. Lindenberger, *Streams from the Valley of Berachah* (New York: Christian Alliance, 1893); and Sarah Freeman Mix, *The Life of Mrs. Edward Mix, Written by Herself in 1880 with Appendix* (Torrington, CT: Press of the Register Printing Co., 1884).

periodicals for the express purpose of propagating the doctrines and practices of healing through faith. The movement's interdenominational character and widespread popularity became apparent in June of 1885, when over fifteen hundred representatives from at least nine countries gathered in London for an "International Conference on Divine Healing and True Holiness."[23]

Although faith cure and Christian Science developed independently and remained largely unaware of one another throughout the 1870s, tensions between their leaders escalated during the early 1880s. As public interest in spiritual healing increased, competition for converts intensified. The tendency of many observers and even some participants to conflate Christian Science and faith cure caused consternation among proponents on both sides and prompted apologists to clarify the boundaries that separated practitioners of Eddy's "metaphysical" mind cure from those who embraced divine healing through "the prayer of faith." In 1885, the growing antagonism between these two movements came to a head when A. J. Gordon, one of the leading apologists for faith cure, published an open letter condemning Christian Science as "a system of spiritual malpractice" that propagated "false doctrines," "bad religious teaching," and insidious "delusion." While he admitted that practitioners of Christian Science were "effecting some marked cures," Gordon claimed that these recoveries involved "an occult principle of healing" that led unsuspecting subjects "away from the simple faith of the Gospel into a vague and transcendental misbelief."[24]

Eddy rebutted Gordon's accusations in a public address delivered in Boston's Tremont Temple and later reiterated her defense in a variety of journal articles and tracts. Not only did Gordon misrepresent Christian Science, Eddy proclaimed, he misunderstood her philosophy of healing completely. In fact, she asserted, a thorough examination of *Science and Health* would prove that Christian Science was superior to the theory and practice of faith cure that Gordon espoused. Christian Science healing, Eddy argued, "is not a remedy of faith alone, but combines faith with understanding." Advocates of divine healing, Eddy suggested, promoted "blind belief" in the biblical promises without encouraging petitioners to comprehend the deeper truth of "metaphysical healing" to which these promises pointed. "Metaphysical or divine science," she

---

23. *Record of the International Conference on Divine Healing and True Holiness Held at the Agricultural Hall, London, June 1 to 5, 1885* (London: J. Snow and Co. and Bethshan, 1885). For a fuller account of these developments, see Curtis, *Faith in the Great Physician*.

24. Gordon's open letter originally appeared in *The Congregationalist* in the spring of 1885 and was subsequently reprinted as a tract in numerous periodicals. Citations in this essay are taken from A. J. Gordon, "'Christian Science' Tested by Scripture," *Triumphs of Faith* (December 1886): 276–80.

explained in a sermon entitled "Christian Healing," "reveals the Principle and method of perfection, — how to attain a mind in harmony with God, in sympathy with all that is right and opposed to all that is wrong, and a body governed by this mind."[25]

Despite her disputes with proponents of faith cure regarding the nature of Christian Science and the proper philosophy and practice of healing, Eddy recognized that she shared common cause with these adversaries when it came to the challenge of combating scientific naturalism, philosophical materialism, and religious skepticism. In a pamphlet intended to lay out the differences between Christian Science and divine healing, Eddy emphasized one important point of accord. Both movements, she argued, affirmed that "God is not unable or unwilling to heal" in the modern era. Even she and A. J. Gordon, her most vocal opponent, could agree that the promises of healing contained in the Bible remained in effect in the present, Eddy suggested. Expressing her approval of Gordon's assertion that "The prayer of faith shall save the sick, and it is doing it to-day; and as the faith of the Church increases, and Christians more and more learn their duty to believe all things written in the Scriptures, will such manifestations of God's power increase among us," Eddy declared that "such sentiments" were consistent with Christian Science. In both cases, healing represented a hearty riposte to doubting skeptics by proving that prayer put suffering petitioners in touch with a living and active God who possessed authority over all nature and who desired to supply "all human needs."[26]

Neither A. J. Gordon nor any of his colleagues in the divine healing movement ever publicly acknowledged Christian Science as an ally in the struggle against naturalism and skepticism. The strategies that advocates of faith cure employed against rising agnosticism, however, did closely resemble those that Christian Scientists adopted. Like Eddy, proponents of faith cure lamented the "materialism and infidelity" of the modern era and argued that healing represented a "protest" against these insidious ideologies. In his influential work, *The Ministry of Healing: or, Miracles of Cure in All Ages*, Gordon argued that instances of physical recovery through the prayer of faith stood as a bulwark against the corrosive tides of contemporary culture. The "gracious deliverance" of a con-

25. Mary Baker Eddy, "Defence of Christian Science against Rev. Joseph Cook and Dr. A. J. Gordon's Religious Ban," *Journal of Christian Science* 2, no. 16 (March 1885): 1–2; "A Strong Reply," *Christian Science Journal* 3, no. 1 (April 1885): 5; *Christian Science: No and Yes*; *Retrospection and Introspection* (Boston: W. G. Nixon, 1891), 54; and Mrs. Glover [Mary Baker] Eddy, *Christian Healing: A Lecture Delivered at Boston* (1886; repr., Cambridge: John Wilson and Son University Press, 1906), 13.

26. Eddy, *Christian Science: No and Yes*, 41.

sumptive from the "edge of the grave" or the instantaneous cure of an opium addict whose habit had "baffled for years every device of the physician" — these kinds of exhibitions of divine power, Gordon contended, proved that God was ever at work in the world, and thus helped to shore up the faltering faith of wavering Christians against the "indignant clamor of the skeptics."[27]

Many champions of faith cure shared Gordon's confidence that modern displays of divine healing could help contemporary Christians defend against the pernicious philosophies of "this present evil age." Experiences of bodily restoration, argued Gordon and associates such as A. B. Simpson, offered empirical evidence of God's existence and ongoing activity in contrast to the pervasive naturalism that characterized much of late nineteenth-century scientific inquiry. "Who can tell but God may have chosen these very manifestations of His power upon human bodies, in this material age," one writer queried, "to answer the unbelief of science, and speak more loudly than all our learned lecturers for His eternal power and Godhead?" Those who insisted that God healed only through "causes, effects, means, second causes, and the order of nature," Simpson contended, constructed "a little fence" around God and refused to allow God "to step out of the enclosure for a moment, or the poor sufferer even to reach Him through the bars." According to this framework, God became "a prisoner in His own world," and "His poor children" could not "get at Him except through the official red tape of the old economy of nature and law." Recent instances of miraculous healing shattered this stifling system, Simpson asserted, by proving that God's Holy Spirit could not be confined by the rules of cause and effect or the dictates of human logic. "Blessed be His Holy Name," Simpson exclaimed, "the resurrection of Jesus Christ from the dead has burst the iron bars of mere natural law, and given us a living Lord." This living Christ, Simpson suggested, continued to intervene in the world in a supernatural manner, making his presence manifest in the spiritual lives and "mortal flesh" of faithful believers.[28]

Against the growing sway of scientific materialism, miraculous cures testified to the reality of a personal, transcendent, yet ever-present deity who overrode the seemingly inviolable laws of nature in response to petitionary prayer. And they did so, their defenders argued, in keeping with the "scientific method" of "rigid induction." In this view, accounts of divine healing represented verifiable data of the kind demanded by the most rigorous empiricist. Whereas spiritual

27. Gordon, *Ministry of Healing*, 1–13.

28. Gordon, *Ministry of Healing*, 2; "For Us, or for the Apostles?," *The Word, Work and World* 1 (July 1882): 245; and A. B. Simpson, "The Gospel of Healing; Divine Healing and Demonism Not Identical. A Protest and Reply to Dr. Buckley in the Century Magazine. Concluded," *The Word, Work and World* 7 (August 1886): 114–22.

experiences such as conversion or sanctification could be "deceptive and difficult to interpret," Gordon maintained, physical cures provided tangible, observable proof of the Holy Spirit's ongoing and supernatural activity. "This is a kind of testimony," Gordon asserted, "which is not easily ruled out of court."[29]

Indeed, advocates of faith cure argued that instances of miraculous physical healing had proliferated in the latter decades of the nineteenth century precisely because skeptical scientists such as Tyndall were demanding empirical evidence to prove that God intervened in the realm of nature in response to intercessory prayer on behalf of the sick. "Have you ever noticed," A. B. Simpson inquired at the International Conference on Divine Healing in 1885, "that ever since the hour when Professor Tyndal [*sic*] . . . challenged the world for an example of faith, God has taken hold of this thing in the most marvellous manner. He has covered the world with answers to Scepticism." The Reverend D. D. Smith, another delegate at the gathering, made a similar point. "Twenty years ago, Professor Tyndal [*sic*] proposed . . . to make a challenge to the Christian world to test the power of prayer," Smith proclaimed. "The Christian church was then afraid to accept the challenge, but I doubt whether he could make it to-day. I think it would be answered by the testimonies in this place. I think we should have sufficient evidence to show that prayer is a power, a force, an answer — sufficient to prove that Christ is a Saviour of the body as well as the soul."[30]

In addition to countering the challenges of scientists who cried out "against 'the dogma of divine interference,'" demonstrations of miraculous healing, proponents argued, also undermined the claims of theologians who maintained that God had ceased to work in a supernatural manner after the apostolic era. According to many nineteenth-century Protestants, and particularly those who participated in the Calvinist tradition, Jesus had performed miracles such as healing the sick in order to reveal his divinity. Once the Christian church had been established, supernatural signs were no longer necessary. The age of miracles had ceased with the apostles, in this view, and although it was still permissible to pray for relief from suffering, Christians should expect God to heal them through natural agencies, or "secondary causes," rather than through a supernatural act of divine power.[31]

Critics of this view such as A. J. Gordon argued that "cessationism," com-

---

29. Robert L. Stanton, "Healing Through Faith," *The Presbyterian Review* 5 (1884): 51; Gordon, *Ministry of Healing*, 175.

30. *Record of the International Conference*, 69, 92.

31. Mullin's *Miracles* offers a thorough account of both Protestant and Catholic attitudes toward miracles and particularly toward claims of miraculous healing leading up to and during the nineteenth century. Chapter 4, "The Question of Healing," 83–107, is especially useful.

bined with assaults upon the reliability of Scripture from the new higher criticism, had caused the church to "drift into an unseemly cautiousness toward the miraculous." Even "true hearted and sincere" Christians, Gordon lamented, were "in danger of being frightened out of their faith in the supernatural" as the result of a growing skepticism regarding the authenticity of biblical miracles and the stubborn tendency of "traditionalist" theologians to inveigh against contemporary instances of divine intervention. Against these two enemies of faith, Gordon and his colleagues argued, modern manifestations of God's supernatural healing power proved the veracity of the scriptural miracles while simultaneously refuting what A. B. Simpson dubbed the "spirit of . . . cold traditional theological rationalism" that characterized liberal Unitarians, Calvinist Presbyterians, and other Protestants who insisted that "the day of miracles was over."[32]

Cessationism and higher criticism were also troubling to Christian Scientists. Like advocates of faith cure, Eddy and her followers censured skeptics who doubted the accounts of healing contained in the Bible and reprimanded theologians who claimed that "healing the sick by the power of divine Spirit is not permissible in these days, *because the age of miracles is past.*" According to Christian Scientists, however, "signs and wonders of healing power" — those performed by Jesus as well as modern instances of physical recovery — were not "abnormal or miraculous." "Christian Science," wrote one proponent, "does not believe in miracles, as such. . . . We believe the events recorded in the Bible took place, but we insist that they were not miraculous, — that is, outside the lawful, divine order of events, — but that they were in full accord with spiritual law — the law which not only Jesus himself fulfilled, but which he expected his followers to fulfill *always*, to the end of time, in salvation from both sin and sickness." Experiences of healing, another author maintained, were "the outcome of a mental power over matter which belongs to all spirituality, and is in accord with a law which is as universal as gravitation." Through her "great discovery" of Christian Science, Eddy explained, "the miracles in the Bible, which had before seemed to me supernatural, grew divinely natural and apprehensible; though uninspired interpreters ignorantly pronounce Christ's healing miraculous, instead of seeing therein the operation of the divine law." By reinterpreting miracles of healing as simultaneously natural and divine events, Christian Scientists appealed to the

32. Gordon, *Ministry of Healing*, esp. 1–13; A. B. Simpson, "The Gospel of Healing," *The Word, Work and World* 3 (April 1883): 57–60; and F. P. Church to Charles Cullis, July 16, 1884, in *Other Faith Cures; or Answers to Prayer in the Healing of the Sick*, ed. Charles Cullis (Boston: Willard Tract Repository, 1885), 137–38.

culturally authoritative rhetoric of science in order to refute biblical critics, traditionalist theologians, and scientific materialists who denied that contemporary cures represented displays of "God's presence and power."[33]

Although staunch skeptics like Tyndall remained dubious about claims of healing — whether described as "modern miracles" or demonstrations of "metaphysical Science" — many late nineteenth-century Protestants accepted accounts of physical restoration through the prayer of faith or Christian Science as empirical proof of God's willingness and ability to conquer sickness and pain in the present era. Throughout the 1880s, beneficiaries of Christian Science and divine healing composed narratives describing remarkable recoveries from all sorts of distressing ailments and disabling diseases. Untold numbers of these testimonials appeared in popular religious newspapers, in widely circulated anthologies, and in periodicals established for the express purpose of promoting divine healing or Christian Science. Others recited their stories at conventions, camp meetings, and church services. By the thousands, people of all ages, socioeconomic classes, denominational backgrounds, and geographical regions of the United States, Britain, and Europe professed to have been cured from boils and blindness; from catarrh and cancer; from dyspepsia and drug addiction; from fevers and "female complaints"; from headaches and heart disease; in short, from all manner of illnesses ranging from seemingly minor maladies to life-threatening afflictions, and from ostensibly nervous or psychogenic disorders to infirmities that were obviously organic in nature. Surely experiences like these established the efficacy of prayer on behalf of the sick and the legitimacy of spiritual healing, their patrons asserted. What better evidence could empiricists ask for?

The Hermeneutics of Healing:
Scientific Empiricism versus Spiritual Discernment

Much to the chagrin of Christian Scientists and proponents of faith cure, accounts of metaphysical and miraculous healing failed to convince many committed critics that prayer made any difference in the process of physical recovery or that God was actively involved in restoring the sick to health. The most

---

33. "Answers to Questions," *Journal of Christian Science* 2, no. 12 (November 1884): 2–3; "When did Miracles Cease?," *Christian Science Journal* 4, no. 7 (October 1886): 176–77; Margaret Ford Moran, "Metaphysical Healing," *Christian Science Journal* 5, no. 2 (May 1887): 74–79; "Christian Science Mind-Healing *versus* Medical Missions," *Christian Science Journal* 5, no. 10 (March 1888): 638; "The Methodist Review," *Christian Science Journal* 4, no. 1 (April 1886): 24; and Eddy, *Retrospection and Introspection*, 24.

cynical detractors accused Christian Science practitioners and divine healing advocates of perpetrating fraud and quackery, while lamenting the gullibility and ignorance of those who sought help from these supposed charlatans. The Reverend Samuel T. Spear, a trained physician and Presbyterian minister, contended that most cases of faith cure were "the products of imposture, or the product of delusion, or of both combined." In an article entitled "Divine Healing," published in *Science*, C. F. Nichols, a medical doctor, dubbed "'Divine Healers,' 'Christian Scientists,' 'Faith' and 'Mind Curers' . . . parasites in the medical profession" who propagated "hypocritical nonsense" and catered to "the childish credulity" of their patients.[34]

Other skeptics argued that participants in spiritual healing movements were sincere but misguided. The recoveries effected through Christian Science and faith cure may have involved genuine experiences of physical healing, these critics contended, but these instances of bodily improvement could usually, if not always, be explained without appeal to supernatural or metaphysical activity. "Many of the cases which are ascribed to the miraculous power of faith and prayer are *alike* due to the *vis medicatrix natura*," wrote Presbyterian pastor Marvin Vincent in an essay denouncing divine healing. Methodist minister and Boston University professor Luther T. Townsend made a similar point in his 1885 treatise *"Faith-Work," "Christian Science," and Other Cures*. "It is estimated by medical authorities that nineteen out of twenty people suffering from the ordinary acute diseases, if left to nature, get well," Townsend observed. Drawing upon "modern" theories of "disease and cure," Townsend highlighted the "striking similarity" between the supposedly miraculous healings associated with the faith cure movement and those recoveries "effected by saints' relics, mesmerism, holy wells, touching for 'king's evil,' by 'metallic tractors,' by blue glass, by Prince Hohnlohe, by Jacob the Zouve," as well as by the "so-called allopath, the homeopath, the isopath, the physiopath, the eclectic, the botanic, the cold-water curer, the electrician, the so-termed Christian Scientist." Finding "no essential difference" among the remarkable recoveries ascribed to these various agents, Townsend concluded that the healing power of nature accounted for the vast majority of these cures.[35]

Taking Townsend's argument a step further, some detractors maintained that physical healings allegedly brought about through Christian Science or

34. Samuel T. Spear, "The Faith Cure," *The Independent* 34, no. 14 (September 1882): 7–8; C. F. Nichols, "Divine Healing," *Science* 14, no. 22 (January 1892).

35. Marvin R. Vincent, "Modern Miracles," *The Presbyterian Review* 15 (July 1883): 473–502; and Luther T. Townsend, *"Faith-Work," "Christian Science," and Other Cures* (Boston: W. A. Wilde, 1885), 24–51.

faith cure were, in fact, the result of "mental impressions" or, less charitably, "imagination." The well-known physician William A. Hammond, a former surgeon general of the United States Army and an expert on "nervous diseases," conducted numerous experiments in the increasingly popular field of mental therapeutics, the outcomes of which led him to conclude that all "so-called miracles" of recovery, including "the healing of the sick by the direct interposition of Providence," were the product of "expectant attention or faith." "It is not a matter of the slightest consequence what the thing is in which the faith is put," Hammond maintained. "It makes no difference: one is just as efficacious as the other." Citing similar experiments in "mental physiology," "psychological researches," and "suggestive medicine," Methodist minister James M. Buckley asserted that cures wrought through "faith-healing, Christian Science and kindred phenomena," among which he included animal magnetism, spiritualism, Mormonism, and Roman Catholicism (particularly the miracles reported at Knock Chapel in Ireland and Lourdes in France), were "a natural result of mental or emotional states." All of these movements, Buckley asserted, succeeded in curing certain nervous ailments and sometimes even acute diseases, but they did so not through any particular supernatural or metaphysical claim but rather through the purely natural appeal to the power of suggestion.[36]

While critics like Buckley and Hammond were willing to acknowledge that faith in metaphysics or God's miraculous power frequently produced positive physical effects, other observers were less sanguine about the purported benefits of Christian Science and divine healing. According to some detractors, both Christian Scientists and proponents of faith cure vastly overstated their rates of success. "The fact is," Luther Townsend declared, "that many sick people who apply to our faith-cure establishments are not in the least benefited." A. F. Schauffler made a similar observation: "Let it be well noted, hundreds are not healed at all, who yet want to be healed." For every testimonial that leaders of spiritual-healing movements presented as proof of the value of prayer on

---

36. William H. Hammond, "The Scientific Relations of Modern Miracles," *The International Review* 10 (March 1881): 225–42; and James Monroe Buckley, "Faith-Healing and Kindred Phenomena," *The Century Illustrated Monthly Magazine* 32 (June 1886): 221–36. See also James Monroe Buckley, "Faith-Healing and Kindred Phenomena (Supplementary Article)," *The Century Illustrated Monthly Magazine* 33 (March 1887): 781–87. Both of these articles were reprinted along with two essays on what Buckley considered "kindred phenomena" — "Christian Science and 'Mind-Cure'" and "Dreams, Nightmares and Somnambulism" — as *Faith-Healing, Christian Science and Kindred Phenomena* (New York: Century, 1898).

behalf of the sick, opponents like Townsend and Schauffler argued, numerous incidents of failure went unreported.[37]

Furthermore, critics asserted, the evidence that advocates of faith cure and Christian Science did offer on behalf of their respective theories and practices of healing was inconclusive, if not utterly specious. Many of those "reported as 'cured,'" Schauffler contended, "are not at all 'cured.'" Some, he argued, were merely "benefited" while others experienced relapses. The most troubling cases, in his view, were those who claimed "to be healed of disease even while the 'symptoms' continue." Both Christian Scientists and exponents of divine healing, observers like Schauffler noted, counseled sick persons to believe that God had banished sickness from the body and to act accordingly, regardless of any sensory evidence to the contrary. "Faith-cure folk . . . are taught by their leaders to claim that they are healed as soon as they have been anointed and prayed over, and that in spite of any subsequent symptoms that may remain," Schauffler reported, substantiating his declaration with an example excerpted from "directions to patients, given by a clergyman":

> When anointed, believe that you do now receive, *i.e.*, say, I am healed *now* . . . Believe against contrary to the physical evidence [*sic*]. After having claimed the Promise, be not surprised at the continuance of symptoms and physical pains. You may expect sudden and powerful returns of your sickness after anointings and prayers. But carefully note that they are only tests of your faith. You ought not to recognize any disease, believing that God has rebuked it.[38]

Mary Baker Eddy offered similar advice. "Dismiss the first mental admission that you are sick; dispute sense with science. . . . Not to admit disease, is to conquer it," she counseled her readers in the first edition of *Science and Health*. "When symptoms of sickness are present, meet them with the resistance of mind against matter, and you will control them. . . . Silently or audibly, according to the circumstances, you should dispute the reality of disease."[39]

Statements such as these bewildered many of the skeptics whom Christian Scientists and advocates of divine healing sought to persuade through the presentation of "numerous and marvelous 'cures.'" "We are left in doubt as to the re-

---

37. Townsend, *"Faith-Work," "Christian Science," and Other Cures*, 57; and A. F. Schauffler, "Faith-Cures: A Study in Five Chapters," *Century Magazine* 31 (December 1885): 274–78.

38. Schauffler, "Faith-Cures," 274–78.

39. Mary Baker Glover [Eddy], *Science and Health* (Boston: Christian Scientist, 1875), 396, 453–54.

ality of the cure," Schauffler noted, "by the singular use of language which faith-cure folk employ. . . . Such unwonted use of language staggers ordinary mortals, and makes them wary in receiving testimony from those who allow themselves such liberties." How could proponents of metaphysical and miraculous healing assert that they provided demonstrable proof of prayer's efficacy and God's ability to vanquish sickness in the modern period when the evidence they presented in support of this claim was often imperceptible to the physical senses?[40]

The answers faith-cure exponents and Christian Scientists proposed to this question expose a fundamental tension in their attitudes toward empiricism. On the one hand, they insisted that instances of healing supplied substantiation of prayer's efficacy and confirmation of God's reality, presence, and power in the contemporary era in a manner consistent with the experimental method that characterized modern scientific inquiry. At the same time, however, leaders of these two movements warned against gauging God's healing activity according to scientific standards alone. As an epistemological framework, they suggested, empiricism relied exclusively upon the testimony of the physical senses, and while the data obtained through sensory observation proved useful for verifying the value of prayer on behalf of the sick, it was not sufficient for fully comprehending the spiritual truths to which metaphysical and divine healing bore witness.

Rather than heralding empiricism as an unambiguous harbinger of progress, as scientists such as Tyndall were wont to do, Christian Scientists and proponents of divine healing highlighted the limitations of this approach to knowledge. Those whose purview encompassed only the physical realm, they maintained, failed to perceive the supernatural or metaphysical power through which God promised to restore ailing bodies and reform sinful souls. "Evidence drawn from the five physical senses relates solely to human reason," Mary Baker Eddy declared in *Science and Health*, "and because of opacity to the true light, human reason dimly reflects and feebly transmits Jesus's works and words."[41] Through the study of Christian Science, she contended, individuals cultivated a new faculty of perception that enabled them to "rise above the evidence of the senses and take hold of the eternal evidences of Truth."[42]

Proponents of faith cure stressed the deficiencies of a purely empirical epistemology in a similar fashion. "Sense looks at things *seen*," wrote one apologist for divine healing, "faith looks at 'the things *not seen*,' and works upon the promises

40. Schauffler, "Faith-Cures," 274–78.
41. Eddy, *Science and Health with Key to the Scriptures*, 117.
42. "A Strong Reply," 4–6.

of God as 'the *substance* of things hoped for.'"[43] In order to grasp God's promises of healing, proponents of faith cure argued, ailing sufferers needed to learn to see through the "eyes of faith," rather than relying solely upon the observations of their physical senses to interpret their experiences. "Belief or faith is the *evidence* in our mind of things as yet unseen," wrote Carrie Judd in *The Prayer of Faith*, one of the seminal texts of the divine healing movement. "Before we have the evidence of our senses in regard to the matter, we accept the evidence of faith."[44]

According to Christian Scientists and advocates of faith cure, healing required a profound perceptual reorientation. Sick persons seeking relief from their afflictions had to disregard the "testimony of the physical senses" in order that they might discern the divine truth that lay beyond the flesh. Only by being "transformed by the renewal of [their minds]" could suffering individuals hope to comprehend the power of God that promised to set them free from the diseases that plagued their bodies and the sins that sullied their souls. Leaders of these two movements recognized, however, that overlooking observable or tangible phenomena in a cultural environment that increasingly valued empirical evidence as the primary arbiter of truth was no easy prospect. From their perspective, naturalistic empiricism represented a kind of epistemological captivity that ensnared sick persons within a web of sensory stimuli and bound them to believe and to behave according to the physical appearance and sentient experience of their bodies. In order to break free from the tangle of empirical explanations that fettered both their faith and their flesh, proponents of Christian Science and divine healing argued, individuals could engage in spiritual practices that facilitated the interdependent processes of mental, spiritual, and corporeal transformation.

For those whose consciousness of pain and commitment to an empirical outlook made it difficult to deny the "evidence of the senses" in favor of the "evidence of faith," epistemological reorientation began with prayer. "Prayer," Mary Baker Eddy remarked, "makes new and scientific discoveries of God, of His goodness and power. It shows us more clearly than we saw before, what we already have and are; and most of all, it shows us what God is."[45] Through the practice of prayer, Eddy explained, sufferers learned to "silence the material senses" so that they might perceive the metaphysical truths that would expose the falsehoods of sickness, disease, and death. "To enter into the heart of prayer,"

---

43. Carrie F. Judd, "Faith without Works," *Triumphs of Faith* 4 (October 1884): 145–46.
44. Judd, *Prayer of Faith*, 42.
45. Eddy, *Christian Science: No and Yes*, 39.

Eddy wrote in *Science and Health*, "the door of the erring senses must be closed. Lips must be mute and materialism silent, that man may have audience with the Spirit, the divine Principle, Love, which destroys all error."[46] Silent prayer, in this view, ushered a petitioner into the presence of God, an experience that enabled her to "relinquish material things," "rise above sensuality," and obtain the "advanced spiritual understanding" that reversed "the testimony of the physical senses" and revealed "man as harmoniously existent in Truth, which is the only basis of health."[47]

Advocates of faith cure also commended prayer as a principal means of promoting a reformation of the mental faculties. In a widely circulated article entitled "The 'Look on Jesus,'" for example, pastor Otto Stockmayer (1838–1917), one of the principal advocates of divine healing in Switzerland, exhorted his readers to "contemplate Jesus." Meditating on Christ was necessary, Stockmayer argued, because of contemplation's power to shape perception. "When we fix our eyes upon an object, we put ourselves in contact with it, we place ourselves under its influence, we allow it to act upon our hearts," he explained. "Looking around about us, as well as constantly looking at ourselves, cannot but awaken and nourish evil in us," he continued. "The world which man carries within him . . . as well as the world that surrounds him, keeps him always a captive, he feels himself chained to visible things." Only by setting his sights on Christ could a man gain release from the sensations that imprisoned him. To gaze at Jesus, Stockmayer affirmed, was to look away from one's self and one's surroundings; to focus attention on the eternal, rather than the temporal; to deny the physical in favor of the spiritual.[48]

Contemplating Christ, in other words, reoriented a person's perspective so that certain realities suddenly became visible while other things were obscured from view. As Anna Prosser, one of Carrie Judd's close associates, intoned in her testimony of healing, "Since my eyes were fixed on Jesus, I've lost sight of all beside, so enchained my spirit's vision, looking at the crucified."[49] Prayer, from this perspective, fostered a focus on God that eclipsed tangible experience. When Charles Cullis prayed with a city missionary from Chicago, for example, this woman, who had struggled with sickness for years and who feared that perhaps "faith healing" was "not of sound doctrine," "lost sight of everything save Christ." Doubts disappeared as the "holy ghost was filling me unutterably full,"

46. Eddy, *Science and Health with Key to the Scriptures*, 11, 15.

47. Eddy, *Science and Health*, 3rd rev. ed. (1881), 174; Eddy, *Science and Health with Key to the Scriptures*, 120.

48. Otto Stockmayer, "The 'Look on Jesus,'" *Words of Faith* 11 (August 1885): 93–96.

49. Anna W. Prosser, *From Death to Life: An Autobiography* (Buffalo: McGerald, 1901), 198.

she wrote. The indwelling presence of God, she implied, banished all thoughts of unbelief, as well as her awareness of her physical sufferings: "My bodily ailments were not in my mind. . . . I rose and walked out of the room, downstairs, into the street, and with very little aid seated myself in the carriage."[50]

Mary Mossman, in her autobiography, *Steppings in God; or, the Hidden Life Made Manifest*, made a similar argument about the importance of seeking "a perfect coincidence of the finite mind with the Infinite" through the practice of contemplative prayer. In order to "receive the manifestation of healing," Mossman suggested, we must "pass on into deeper spiritual life and affiliate more with the Divine mind concerning us." When our minds are brought into agreement with God's mind, she explained, "we no longer see the old man with its fleshly desires and diseases, but the new man created in Jesus Christ, and in the new life which we by faith receive we press on to apprehend all that for which we are apprehended of Christ Jesus. . . . Receiving life and light from this higher plane, we lose sight of material things." Although she often "seemed to be very ill," Mossman insisted that by "seeing *Jesus only*," she was able to disregard the feelings of her flesh, concentrating instead upon "wonderful manifestations of God's loving care."[51]

Through the practice of prayer, proponents of Christian Science and divine healing contended, sick persons trained their minds to focus on spiritual realities rather than sensory suffering. Engaging in contemplative or meditative practices expanded an individual's ability to discern the workings of God in both soul and body, even if this divine activity remained imperceptible to the physical senses. Leaders of both movements contended that cultivating this capacity to comprehend metaphysical or supernatural truths was essential to the curative process. By claiming the divine purposes and promises made manifest through prayer, ailing sufferers could declare themselves cured despite any and all sensory indications to the contrary.

Both Christian Scientists and exponents of faith cure maintained that, in most cases, the body would ultimately bear witness to the spiritual realities perceived through "eyes of faith." Those who persistently held "in mind only the perfect model" of health through the practice of prayer, Eddy asserted, would eventually destroy the "evidence of the senses." "Argue down those witnesses against your peace," she counseled, "and you will destroy those witnesses, and the disease will disappear."[52] Advocates of faith cure made similar recommen-

---

50. S. G. C., "My Help and My Deliverer," *Triumphs of Faith* 1 (October 1881): 153–57.

51. Mossman, *Steppings in God*, 17–22, 25, 110–19.

52. Eddy, *Science and Health*, 3rd rev. ed. (1881), 186.

dations. "Accept the truth of your healing accomplished long ago on Calvary's cross, and in God's own time (perhaps very quickly) the evidence of your senses will be added to that of your faith," one spokesperson proclaimed.[53] Carrie Judd put it this way: "We are to believe that the blessing prayed for is ours solely on the assurance of God's word, without any reference to the apparent state of things . . . and then in God's own time . . . we shall have that possession made manifest to our human sense as well as to our faith."[54] Although they admitted that, in some cases, pain and signs of illness might linger for a very long time — perhaps even until a person's death — leaders like Judd and Eddy insisted that the spiritual would ultimately triumph over the material. In the meantime, they argued, those who learned to "look not to the things that are seen but to the things that are unseen" through the practice of prayer could grasp "the reality" of metaphysical or divine healing that lay "back of and below all symptoms."[55]

Conclusion

For late nineteenth-century American and British Protestants who took part in Christian Science and faith cure, divine healing entailed the development of spiritual discernment through the practice of devotional disciplines such as contemplation, meditation, and prayer. By cultivating the capacity to interpret their experiences according to distinctive theological frameworks, participants in these movements learned to define healing in a manner that encompassed a broader range of meanings than those proffered under the rubric of scientific empiricism. Although proponents of Christian Science and faith cure insisted that instances of metaphysical or miraculous healing provided demonstrable evidence against naturalism, materialism, and skepticism, they simultaneously questioned the value of the scientific method for ascertaining spiritual phenomena. Discerning the process of spiritual healing, in their view, called for a more holistic epistemology — a perspective that enabled petitioners to discount the evidence of the senses in favor of the evidence of faith.

Hermeneutics thus lay at the heart of late nineteenth-century debates over the meaning and experience of spiritual or divine healing. Then, as now, par-

53. Prosser, *From Death to Life*, 127–28.
54. Carrie F. Judd, "Faith's Reckonings," *Triumphs of Faith* 1 (January 1881): 1–4.
55. A. B. Simpson, "The Gospel of Healing," *Triumphs of Faith* 3 (November 1883): 257–60.

ticular epistemological commitments shaped the ways in which believers and skeptics, scientists and theologians, physicians and sufferers approached and understood the problem of sickness and the pursuit of health. In recent decades, disputes over how to define, measure, and interpret the phenomenon of spiritual healing have proliferated and intensified as both medical researchers and religious persons from a variety of faith traditions have endeavored to enumerate the connections between faith or spirituality and physical, mental, and emotional well-being. Studies intended to assess the value of meditative practices for coping with pain or to test efficacy of prayer for curing bodily illness have fostered vigorous and often contentious deliberations among scientists, theologians, ethicists, medical professionals, and lay people that echo, in many respects, late nineteenth-century responses to Tyndall's "prayer-gauge" proposal. Some contemporary proponents of faith healing, like their predecessors in the divine healing movement, have suggested that prayer studies will provide empirical evidence of God's existence and ability to intervene in the natural world. Other believers worry that applying empirical methods to matters of faith violates the ineffable character of religion. Scientific detractors complain that both the questions posed and the techniques employed in these experiments are insufficiently rigorous. Still other observers protest that the definitions of spirituality employed in most research efforts mask significant theological distinctions among religious traditions and in so doing fail to take into account the particular ways in which people of different faiths interpret illness and respond to bodily discomfort.[56]

56. For overviews of studies that attempt to chart the connection between religious faith, spiritual practice, and health or healing, see Candy Gunther Brown, *Testing Prayer: Science and Healing* (Cambridge, MA: Harvard University Press, 2012); Harold G. Koenig and Harvey J. Kohen, eds., *The Link between Religion and Health: Psychoneuroimmunology and the Faith Factor* (New York: Oxford University Press, 2002); Harold G. Koenig, Michael E. McCullough, and David B. Larson, *Handbook of Religion and Health: A Century of Research Reviewed* (New York: Oxford University Press, 2001); Harold G. Koenig, *The Healing Power of Faith: Science Explores Medicine's Last Great Frontier* (New York: Simon & Schuster, 1999); Harold G. Koenig, *Faith and Mental Health: Religious Resources for Healing* (Philadelphia: John Templeton Foundation Press, 2005); and Larry Dossey, *Reinventing Medicine: Beyond Mind-Body to a New Era of Healing* (San Francisco: Harper, 1999). One of the most prominent and tenacious proponents of a positive correlation between spiritual practice and health is Herbert Benson, whose work, *The Relaxation Response* (New York: Morrow, 1975), helped pioneer studies of prayer and well-being. See also Herbert Benson, *Beyond the Relaxation Response: How to Harness the Healing Power of Your Personal Beliefs* (New York: Times, 1984); and Herbert Benson, *Timeless Healing: The Power and Biology of Belief* (New York: Scribner, 1996). For a critique of Benson and other works of this genre, see Sarah Coakley and Kay

In any case, the fervor that characterizes current discussions about the intersections among religious belief, medical science, and healing highlights the central importance of hermeneutics in the therapeutic process. By analyzing how Protestants in an earlier historical period struggled to defend, define, and discern divine healing, this essay has endeavored to put contemporary conversations into broader perspective and to provide a wider frame for thinking about the implications of recent scientific attempts to assess "the value of prayer on behalf of the sick."

Shelemay, eds., *Pain and Its Transformations: The Interface of Biology and Culture* (Cambridge, MA: Harvard University Press, 2007), esp. 77–100, 133–38.

Part Two

What Science Shows Us

4

Meaning in the Neural Investigation of Pain

Howard L. Fields

U p to now in this volume, the specific focus has been on biblical and historical investigation of spiritual healing and its relation to meaning-making in relevant religious communities. But now we turn our focus to modern secular science in order to ask how neuroscience, psychology, and the history and philosophy of science are equipped to conduct themselves in the face of evidences for spiritual healing. In this chapter, the issue of meaning-making and its relation to the neural investigation of pain is put to the fore. And the first thing that strikes us here is a particular *mystery* to be confronted.

Both the religious practitioner and the scientist are of course drawn to mystery. For the religious practitioner, mystery surrounds the metaphysical forces that influence the world, and consequently it is a reservoir of hope and faith. In contrast, the scientist's worldview is neither negated nor supported by the mysterious; rather, mystery is simply unknown and therefore a challenge to be met by experiment and logical analysis. It is the scientist's job to chip away at uncertainty, all the while maintaining faith that a rational, natural (as opposed to supernatural or metaphysical) explanation exists.[1] Thus, it is somewhat risky for the religious practitioner to engage the scientific community in an investigation of bodily healing by faith — submitting their beliefs to rigorous observation, experiment, and proof. Nonetheless, as will be pointed out by Anne Harrington in this volume, empirical studies of healing by prayer are being enthusiastically promoted in some quarters.

---

1. See, for example, Karl Popper, *Objective Knowledge: An Evolutionary Approach* (Oxford: Clarendon, 1972).

Although the published data are still not conclusive, let us assume that rigorous studies do in fact establish a connection between faith and healing. To what end, then? For those who accept either a powerful deity or some other metaphysical force, that observation would be sufficient to show that a cherished religious attitude or practice has a salubrious effect. Others may wish to take the enterprise further by harnessing the scientific method to verify that such a phenomenon has no natural explanation and thereby interpret it as support for their faith in metaphysical forces. In this case, the issue becomes more difficult, and the possibility of finding common ground with the scientific community less likely. To believe in a deity or spiritual agency is one thing, but to invoke such metaphysical constructs to explain phenomena in the natural world throws down the gauntlet to the scientifically inclined. For many scientists, the possibility that faith healing might involve metaphysical forces would arise only if no natural explanations were forthcoming. The challenge for the scientist then is to discover the most likely explanation consistent with the known properties of the natural world. For the scientist, such explanations remove the need for alternative metaphysical explanations. Consequently, the approach taken in this chapter is to focus on the question of how belief per se, independent of its inherent veracity, can produce a therapeutic effect. In other words, regardless of whether such an entity exists, how could the belief in a compassionate deity promote healing? This question is well within the realm of purely scientific inquiry.

The Brain: Meaning, Mind, and Body

Tremendous advances in neuroscience over the past century have revealed a critical truth: our subjective experience of self and the world around us depends on the precise workings of the billions of nerve cells and probably trillions of ever-changing connections between these cells. When these cells are temporarily inactivated, the ongoing stream of conscious experience and behavioral action ceases. Different parts of the brain and their specific connections are necessary for sensory perception, memory, language, and the different appetites (food, procreation, dominance, novelty, and so on) that direct our course through the world. Simply put, the content of our conscious experiences and actions are the result of specific, albeit changeable, patterns of nerve cell activity. This activity is registered in digital pulses called action potentials and in the release of tiny packets of chemical messengers called neurotransmitters.[2] The details of this

2. For more detail, see E. Kandel, T. H. Schwartz, and T. M. Jessell, *Principles of Neural Science*, 5th ed. (New York: Appleton & Lange, 2013).

process are not germane to this discussion, but it is critical to understand that our subjective experience is underlain by neurobiological processes. Changes in our subjective sensations, feelings, and ideas are fundamentally tied to corresponding alterations in neural activity. Although we may not fully understand the nature of the relationship between subjective mental phenomena (mind) and observable brain processes (body), advances in neuroscience have established an intimate link between the two.

In order to appreciate the nature of this link, it is essential to grasp that the operation of the brain is symbolic, by which I mean that it is an organ built to process information about the body and the external world. Its function cannot be understood without studying the tasks that it is built to carry out.[3] The brain is an organ that creates and manipulates *meaning*. Take as an example an object that we see, such as an apple on a table. Reflected light (electromagnetic particles/waves) from the apple reaches our retina where it activates photosensitive pigments that excite retinal neurons in a particular pattern. This pattern reaches our brain through the visual pathways, reaching our cerebral cortex. The neural activity in this pathway is decoded and experienced as "apple." A veridical apple is nowhere to be found in the brain. What is in the brain is a pattern of neural activity (an encoded representation) that means that round, red piece of fruit. Similarly, there is an encoded representation underlying our sense of self and our experience of our own bodies. The mind, the body, and the external world are encoded in different patterns of neural activity. So there is no ontological mind-body problem; mind and body are different arrangements of the same stuff, that is, patterns of neural activity. Since the brain is part of the body and both are objective physical entities, they can interact without the need to postulate any new physical principles. This discovery does not solve the philosophical mind-body problem, but it does require that it be reformulated as a mind-brain problem (i.e., how does brain activity create subjective awareness?). Recognition of the link between brain activity and subjective experience, on the one hand, and between brain activity and bodily function and the experience of the body, on the other, opens up new possibilities of correlating mental phenomena such as belief or faith with a wide range of effects in the physical body. How does this link develop?

In addition to the neural representations activated by sensory stimuli, cumulative changes in the brain occur in an individual's lifetime. One result of this is the development of an individual's personal narrative, a life story that confers a more cohesive level of meaning on the stream of experience. From

3. See, for example, P. Glimcher, *Decisions, Uncertainty, and the Brain: The Science of Neuroeconomics* (Cambridge, MA: MIT Press, 2003).

the standpoint of neuroscience, personal narratives and the beliefs that they include are complex cognitive patterns that have both genetic and environmental causes. They require a sufficiently complex central nervous system, which is the product of our evolutionary and embryonic development. The human brain has distinct cortical regions that are highly specialized for abstract thought, including language (the specificity referred to by Jeeves, chapter 5). However, full development of these capabilities involves learning through personal experience and through exposure to the ideas of other people, received directly or through various media. Although the human brain is well developed at birth, it continues to grow for decades in both size and the complexity of its connections. This growth is guided to a significant degree by associative learning. For example, we learn to associate sounds with physical objects like the barking of a dog, or the sound of a door closing. More abstractly, we also learn to make sounds that can indicate things — that is, we give names to things. At an even more abstract level, we can use sounds to refer to actions (run, carry, bring). Once we have sounds to indicate objects and actions, we can combine them to communicate our needs. Visual symbols can be used to represent things (for example, pictographs, like hieroglyphics) or sounds (words). With auditory or written symbols for objects and actions, people can communicate with each other about possibilities. Furthermore, with written language and the internet, ideas can be communicated across time and space.

All types of learning, including learning a language, involve relatively simple changes in the strength of particular connections between the neurons that already exist in the brain (the plasticity referred to by Jeeves in chapter 5). What happens over time is the development of representations, which are specific groups of neurons that have become interconnected either by genetic programming or by learning. Each individual has a brain that uniquely reflects their genetics and personal life history. As each new situation is approached by individuals, they need to call on their previous experience to select the most appropriate action. This involves making predictions about the cost of the action and the value and probability of the outcome of the action. Much of the human frontal cortex is involved in making these types of decisions.[4] Over time, the iterative process of prediction, action, outcome, learning, and so on leads to a set of memories and to expectations, habits, and opinions. This is a part of the personal narrative, and it is encoded in the pattern of connections in the brain. In many people, this narrative includes the idea of a deity capable of healing

4. See S. M. McClure, D. I. Laibson, G. Loewenstein, and J. D. Cohen, "Separate Neural Systems Value Immediate and Delayed Monetary Rewards," *Science* 306 (2004): 503-7.

directly — that is, it effects a spiritual healing as indicated throughout this volume. Regardless of whether such healings do indeed occur, one can objectively approach the question of how the *belief* in such a healing could promote bodily healing (the spiritual dimensions of healing). The idea of an active deity is based upon (or at least mediated by) a neural representation and, in that way, has a physical basis that is similar to the ideas of self and world. These representations can interact because they have a physically similar code (neural activity) and the neurons have convergent connectivity. For example, if I am very ill and I pray for a speedy recovery, I may have a strong belief that I will recover (which could be based on previous experience or on my interpretation of information from a source I trust and respect — a book, the internet, or a person). This information enhances my expectation that I shall improve. One could say that the neural computation of the future outcome now results in a prediction that the probability of recovery is greater (or that the probability of worsening is lower). This prediction is experienced as an expectation for recovery.

It is likely that the anticipation of benefit or harm depends upon activity in the anterior cingulate cortex.[5] Activity in these neurons can alter activity in the hypothalamus, which controls the pituitary gland and the autonomic nervous system. Through these connections, changes in expectations can lead to changes in bodily function. Activity in cingulate neurons can also lead to activation of brainstem neurons that control pain (see below), so the belief-based expectation of healing will lower pain and produce the experience of improvement. In other words, the neural representation experienced as an expectation of improvement changes the neural representation that gives rise to the symptom of the disease (in this case pain).

Thus, to the extent that the neural underpinnings of belief can be plausibly linked to the neural antecedents of healing, a biological connection between faith and healing becomes a scientifically tractable issue. Focusing on the neural activity that is correlated with mental phenomena obviates the age-old problem of explaining how something mental (for example, faith) could affect one's physical state. Rather, the question concerns whether robust neural control of a given bodily phenomenon (for example, disease remission) can be demonstrated, and to what extent the neural activity underlying a given mental

5. See O. Devinsky, M. J. Morrell, and B. A. Vogt, "Contributions of Anterior Singulate Cortex to Behavior," *Brain* 118 (1995): 279–306; A. Ploghaus, I. Tracey, J. S. Gati, S. Clare, R. S. Menon, P. M. Matthews, and J. N. Rawlins, "Dissociating Pain from Its Anticipation in the Human Brain," *Science* 284 (1999): 1979–81; and M. Shidara and B. J. Richmond, "Anterior Cingulate: Single Neuronal Signals Related to Degree of Reward Expectancy," *Science* 296 (2002): 1709–11.

phenomenon (such as faith) might be involved. One neuroscientific explanation of faith healing would be that it begins with one pattern of neural activity underlying the experience of illness and another underlying the *expectation* of a spiritual cure. The pattern of neural activity underlying the expectation of a cure then causes beneficial changes in the body. But is there any evidence supporting such an explanation?

Placebo Pain Relief: Expectancy, Meaning, and Modulatory Control

Nowhere has the relationship between mental state, neural activity, and healing been studied more extensively than in the area of bodily pain. It has been conclusively demonstrated that one's mental attitude — that is, *what one expects to experience* — has a robust influence on the degree of pain reported when the body is stimulated.[6] The placebo analgesic effect is a well-known example of this phenomenon. For example, if subjects are trained with an infusion of morphine, a subsequent infusion of an inert solution (salt water) that they believe is morphine can dramatically reduce their reported pain. Brain imaging in subjects with robust placebo analgesia confirms these subjective reports by showing reduced activity in the brain areas normally activated by painful stimuli. In addition, other brain areas, including those activated by the powerful pain killer morphine, show increased activity.[7] Finally, the analgesic effect of placebo can be reversed by a molecule that blocks the brain's receptor for opioids.[8] Clearly, the *meaning* of the words ("this is a powerful analgesic") and the *meaning* of the visual stimuli (white coat, syringe, intravenous infusion) combine to induce a state of expectancy for reduced pain. The pattern of neuronal activity underlying this expectancy state involves the release of an endogenous opioid-like substance that acts at the same molecular target as the pain-killing drug morphine.

6. See Luana Colloca and Fabrizio Benedetti, "Placebos and Painkillers: Is Mind as Real as Matter?," *Nature Reviews Neuroscience* 6 (2005): 545–52; and V. Hoffman, A. Harrington, and H. L. Fields, "Pain and the Placebo: What We Have Learned," *Perspectives in Biology and Medicine* 48 (2005): 248–65. Also see, in this regard, the edited volume by Anne Harrington, *The Placebo Effect: An Interdisciplinary Exploration* (Cambridge, MA: Harvard University Press, 1999).

7. F. Eippert, U. Bingel, E. D. Schoell, J. Yacubian, R. Klinger, J. Lorenz, and C. Büchel, "Activation of the Opioidergic Descending Pain Control System Underlies Placebo Analgesia," *Neuron* 63 (2009): 533–43.

8. J. D. Levine, N. C. Gordon, and H. L. Fields, "The Mechanism of Placebo Analgesia," *Lancet* 23 (1978): 654–57.

The research literature on placebo analgesia demonstrates that the level of certainty that one has received an active pain-relieving drug is directly correlated with its pain-relieving power.[9] I would argue that it is precisely in the degree of expectation for recovery that religious belief or faith potentially exerts its greatest healing effect by fostering confidence that there will be a positive outcome. One could imagine the potentially powerful expectancy state induced in a devout individual by the combination of religious belief, prayer, ritual, and the words or touch of a venerable religious leader. While the outcome of healing due to this expectancy state is scientifically tractable, the pathways leading to this state go beyond the biological and include historical, religious, social, and personal factors that contribute to that person's individual narrative as well as the current contextual factors that influence his or her faith in recovery.

Psyche and Soma: How Does the Brain Influence the Body?

While marveling at the placebo (or more generally, expectation-based) analgesic effect, some dismiss its importance to bodily healing because pain is a subjective experience. They argue that pain is subjective and secondary to the disease process so that reducing it does not really represent healing, because the bodily process causing the pain is not necessarily improved. In other words, it is "virtual" healing. However, if one accepts that the brain is a physical entity and is part of the body, this point of view makes little sense. The use of functional imaging has brought pain into the objective world of neural processes. With functional imaging, it is possible to visualize evidence of the neural activity produced by noxious stimuli — that is, the neural representation of pain.[10] Furthermore, as one begins to appreciate the extent to which neural activity controls a variety of bodily functions, the range of phenomena mediated by belief, faith, or spiritual practice that can be explained on the basis of well-established biological principles expands vastly.

Can a change in neural activity lead to bodily healing? The literature on objectively measurable bodily changes caused by expectancy or placebo admin-

9. See A. Pollo, M. Amanzio, A. Arslanian, C. Casadio, G. Maggi, and F. Benedetti, "Response Expectancies in Placebo Analgesia and Their Clinical Relevance," *Pain* 93 (2001): 77–84. Also see Sarah Coakley and Kay Kaufman Shelemay, eds., *Pain and Its Transformations: The Interface of Biology and Culture* (Cambridge, MA: Harvard University Press, 2007).

10. T. D. Wager, L. Y. Atlas, M. A. Lindquist, M. Roy, C. W. Woo, and E. Kross, "An fMRI-Based Neurologic Signature of Physical Pain," *New England Journal of Medicine* 368, no. 15 (2013): 1388–97.

istration is limited. However, there are well-established channels by which the brain can influence the body. The two main portals for bodily control by the brain are the autonomic and endocrine systems. Through these portals, the brain can control the cardiovascular system, the immune system, and various metabolic processes.

Building on the work of physiologist Walter B. Cannon,[11] the endocrinologist Hans Selye developed the concept of the general adaptation syndrome.[12] This is a general response to stress. The stress can be due to physical exertion, bodily disease (for example, a heart attack or cancer), or emotional stress (a financial setback or the loss of a loved one). The experience of emotional stress requires neural activity; in many cases, this would include the neural activity that underlies the prediction of future harm (or loss of reward). The acute stress response includes changes in the autonomic nervous system, which controls heart rate, body temperature, and blood pressure. There is no question that prolonged elevated blood pressure such as might result from prolonged stress is a significant health risk. In fact, evidence shows that stress reduction, for example, through meditative practice can reduce cardiac illness and prolong life.[13]

Beyond the direct cardiovascular effects, the more lasting and detrimental components of stress are mediated by the hypothalamic-pituitary-adrenal (HPA) axis. The HPA axis regulates glucose metabolism, water and electrolyte balance, and immune function. This likely includes frontal areas of the cerebral cortex that connect to the hypothalamus. The hypothalamus is the critical brain structure that controls the autonomic nervous system. This control is exerted through the sympathetic and parasympathetic nervous systems. In addition, it mediates the endocrine activity that leads to elevations of the adrenal cortical hormone cortisol. Cortisol leads to an elevation of blood sugar, enhanced risk of hypertension, stomach ulcers, and obesity.[14] This indicates that to the extent

11. W. B. Cannon, *The Wisdom of the Body* (New York: W. W. Norton, 1939).

12. See H. Selye, "A Syndrome Produced by Diverse Nocuous Agents," *Nature* 138 (1936): 32, as well as H. Selye, *The Stress of Life* (New York: McGraw Hill, 1956).

13. See, for example, R. H. Schneider, C. N. Alexander, F. Staggers, M. Rainforth, J. W. Salerno, A. Hartz, S. Arndt, V. A. Barnes, and S. I. Nidich, "Long-Term Effects of Stress Reduction on Mortality in Persons > or = 55 Years of Age with Systemic Hypertension," *American Journal of Cardiology* 95 (2005): 1060–64.

14. See D. Gomez-Merino, C. Drogou, M. Chennaoui, E. Tiollier, J. Mathieu, C. Y. Guezennec, "Effects of Combined Stress During Intense Training on Cellular Immunity, Hormones and Respiratory Infections," *Neuroimmunomodulation* 12 (2005): 164–72; and R. Rosmond, M. F. Dallman, and P. Björntorp, "Stress-Related Cortisol Secretion in Men: Relationships with Abdominal Obesity and Endocrine, Metabolic and Hemodynamic Abnormalities," *Journal of Clinical Endocrinology & Metabolism* 83 (1998): 1853–59.

that emotional stress can be relieved by religious practice or belief, there are a variety of possible biologically plausible health benefits.

The hypothalamus also controls immune function through two routes. First, via activation of the HPA, cortisol levels increase. Increased blood cortisol reduces immune function and white-blood-cell counts and enhances the susceptibility of the individual to infection. In addition, the hypothalamus exerts control over the immune system via the autonomic nervous system. One way this occurs is via activation of the vagus nerve. The vagus nerve arises in autonomic control regions of the brainstem, which directly control levels of circulating cytokines. The cytokines in turn control the immune system and regulate the response to injury (see below). This autonomic control exerts very powerful regulation of systems critical for survival. For example, stimulating the vagus nerve leads to the release of the neurotransmitter acetylcholine, which controls cytokines. Through this action, the autonomic nervous system promotes the survival of animals exposed to chemical injury that induces a state of cardiovascular collapse.[15]

There is a growing literature supporting the theory of the importance of emotions on the bodily response to disease. In a very telling study, a group of individuals was tested for recent life stresses and then given a standard mixture of mild respiratory viruses.[16] Those who reported a greater level of emotional stress had a significantly greater probability of developing an upper respiratory illness. A more recent study found that a cognitive-behavioral stress reduction program significantly improved immune function as measured by T-cell counts in HIV-infected gay men.[17] A more direct test of psychological control of immune function is provided by the phenomenon of conditioned immunosuppression. As with analgesia, immune suppression can be induced in individuals by behavioral conditioning. Following a training period in which subjects received immunosuppressive drugs plus a flavored drink, the drink alone induced measurable

15. See V. A. Pavlov, M. Ochani, M. Gallowitsch-Puerta, K. Ochani, J. M. Huston, C. J. Czura, Y. Al-Abed, and K. J. Tracey, "Central Muscarinic Cholinergic Regulation of the Systemic Inflammatory Response During Endotoxemia," *Proceedings of the National Academy of the Sciences, USA* 103 (2006): 5219–23.

16. See S. Cohen, D. A. Tyrrell, and A. P. Smith, "Psychological Stress and Susceptibility to the Common Cold," *New England Journal of Medicine* 325 (1991): 606–12.

17. See M. H. Antoni, D. G. Cruess, N. Klimas, K. Maher, S. Cruess, M. Kumar, S. Lutgendorf, G. Ironson, N. Schneiderman, and M. A. Fletcher, "Stress Management and Immune System Reconstitution in Symptomatic HIV-Infected Gay Men Over Time: Effects on Transitional Naive T Cells (CD4+CD45RA+CD29+)," *American Journal of Psychiatry* 159 (2002): 143–45.

immune suppression.[18] Expectancy-based activation of this neural mechanism could lead to remission of a variety of autoimmune diseases, like rheumatoid arthritis, multiple sclerosis, and perhaps rejection of transplanted organs.

Related to actions on immune function, increased levels of perceived stress correlate with reduced rates of wound healing. This effect has been linked to cortisol levels and proinflammatory cytokines.[19] Stress increases cortisol levels and slows the local production of proinflammatory cytokines needed for healing at wound sites. Cytokines are molecules that promote wound healing by attracting inflammatory cells. In a study that explicitly manipulated emotional stress levels, increased levels of stress were associated with a slowed healing of a small skin wound and decreased levels of local cytokine production (IL-6, tumor necrosis factor α, and IL-1β).[20] In fact, these studies of wound healing provide some of the most robust examples of the effect of nervous-system activity on bodily healing. It appears that the neural activity that generates the subject's sense of emotional distress leads to autonomic, endocrine, and immune responses that can either promote disease or healing.

One of the most threatening of diseases is cancer. Many cancers are subject to at least limited control by hormones or the immune system, suggesting a possible link to emotional stress. On the other hand, the question of whether behavioral interventions affect cancer survival is still open. Some studies have provided evidence linking mental state to survival, while others have found no significant effect.[21] It would be extraordinarily interesting for cancer sufferers

18. See M. U. Goebel, A. E. Trebst, J. Steiner, Y. F. Xie, M. S. Exton, S. Frede, A. E. Canbay, M. C. Michel, U. Heemann, M. Schedlowski, "Behavioral Conditioning of Immunosuppression Is Possible in Humans," *FASEB Journal* 16 (2002): 1869–73.

19. On the link to cortisol levels, see, for example, M. Ebrecht, J. Hextall, L. G. Kirtley, A. Taylor, M. Dyson, J. Weinman, "Perceived Stress and Cortisol Levels Predict Speed of Wound Healing in Healthy Male Adults," *Psychoneuroendocrinology* 29 (2004): 798–809. And on proinflammatory cytokines, see J. K. Kiecolt-Glaser, T. J. Loving, J. R. Stowell, W. J. Malarkey, S. Lemeshow, S. L. Dickinson, and R. Glaser, "Hostile Marital Interactions, Proinflammatory Cytokine Production, and Wound Healing," *Archives of the Journal of General Psychiatry* 62 (2005): 1377–84.

20. Note here that IL-6 and IL-1β should be read as "interleukin factor six" and "interleukin factor beta," respectively. Interleukins are intercellular signaling molecules often implicated in immune function and, in this case, increased stress response.

21. See, for example, D. Spiegel, "Effects of Psychotherapy on Cancer Survival," *Nature Reviews Cancer* 2 (2002): 383–89; and P. J. Goodwin, M. Leszcz, M. Ennis, J. Koopmans, L. Vincent, H. Guther, E. Drysdale, M. Hundleby, M. Harvey, M. D. Chochinov, M. Navarro, M. Speca, J. Masterson, L. Dohan, R. Sela, B. Warren, A. Paterson, K. I. Pritchard, A. Arnold, R. Doll, S. E. O'Reilly, G. Quirt, N. Hood, and J. Hunter, "The Effect of Group

if more evidence for the former hypothesis were forthcoming; but, to date, research results are ambiguous.

Summary and Conclusions: Where Is the Mysterious?

In this chapter, I have taken the position that neuroscience is the appropriate discipline to look at for biological explanations of what has been called faith healing. One straightforward possibility is that faith enhances the expectation of a positive outcome. In the area of pain, positive expectation has a robust analgesic effect. Faith can also reduce chronic stress, with a significant effect on the immune system, obesity, and cardiovascular function. Any of these biological actions can influence health and survival. These observations provide a powerful and elegant explanatory core relating spiritual experience to bodily health through well-accepted biological processes. While supporting the beneficial nature of religious faith, these observations do not support metaphysical explanations. To the extent that faith healing is explicable by natural processes, it is difficult to see how demonstrations of the salubrious effect of faith could constitute an argument for metaphysical or divine agency; unless, of course, we broaden our notion of what qualifies as divine.

On the other hand, this neurobiological explanation leaves some significant explanatory gaps to be filled. Foremost among the mysteries that confront neuroscience are the origin and biological function of subjective awareness or consciousness. Consciousness (or mind, in some views) is an emergent property of nervous systems that is not susceptible to direct study using objective methods. In this sense, consciousness is still a miraculous phenomenon at the core of our concept of who we are as individuals and what it means to be alive and human. Like the universe before the big bang and the origin of life, consciousness remains shrouded in mystery.[22]

Psychosocial Support on Survival in Metastatic Breast Cancer," *New England Journal of Medicine* 345 (2001): 1719–26.

22. For more on issues of consciousness and healing, see chapters 5 and 7 in this volume, by Malcolm Jeeves and Philip Clayton, respectively.

5

The Brain and Cognitive Processes in Healing

Malcolm Jeeves

S arah Coakley helpfully reminds us that *spirituality* has become so vogue, yet so vague, a word that it is vital that its meaning be clarified in any discussion of its significance for healing.[1] She points out that for some, spirituality has become an oppositional alternative to institutional or doctrinal religion, often characterized by emotionally satisfying experiential dimensions. Coakley also points out that in this book, we need to be clear whether we are speaking about spiritual healing or the spiritual dimensions of healing. The spiritual dimensions of healing include the beliefs, expectations, and hopes held by an individual and shared within a community of like-minded believers. The focus of what follows is primarily on these spiritual dimensions of healing. Toward the end of the chapter, the evidence reviewed will be set in the context of specific warranted Christian beliefs about the moment-by-moment upholding of a Creator God.

Our starting point may be seen as a response to the prompting by Philip Clayton, who notes that "doubts and objections about spiritual healing might be overcome if one could integrate one's view of spiritual healing with the best current work from within the various relevant sciences."[2] It is to two of the most relevant sciences, psychology and neuroscience, that we look for clues in what follows.

In the spirit of Sarah Coakley's exhortation for semantic hygiene, it is im-

1. See Sarah Coakley, introduction, pp. 4–5.
2. Philip Clayton, chapter 7, p. 141.

portant to make clear that reference to "top-down" processes in what follows is much narrower than that implied by Coakley when she refers to "'top-down' religious 'meaning systems,'" which she puts over against "bottom-up neuroscientific explanations."[3] In this chapter, both "top-down" and "bottom-up" are used primarily within the context of neuropsychological explanations, and only later are they speculatively extended to include "religious 'meaning systems.'" With Coakley, we question the widely held assumption that a belief "has negligible intellectual — let alone neurological or psychological — significance."[4] As Warren Brown has pointed out, "religion may well be a contextual variable that controls the interpretation of the neural events, not a primary outcome of the neural state itself."[5] In discussing research on the neurology of religion, Brown asks, "Would the experience of temporal lobe epileptic discharge be interpreted as religious by a person with no religious background whatsoever?"[6] Brown, in highlighting the relevance of someone's personal beliefs to the way in which the activities in his or her brain are interpreted, hints here at the *embeddedness* of the spiritual dimensions of healing that we shall expand upon later.

The thesis of this chapter, then, will be that the very rapid advances over the last five decades at the interfaces of neuroscience with psychology are potentially most relevant to a fresh understanding of the spiritual dimensions of healing. It has been known for a century and a half that there has been steadily accumulating evidence to show that regions of the brain are selectively specialized for specific abilities. This remarkable *specificity* of function applies both to brain regions and to brain systems. Studies of localization of function within the brain — until relatively recently investigated mainly through bottom-up approaches — have given rise to the widespread belief that there is a fixity about the neural embodiment of cognitive and conceptual abilities. This fixity has frequently been described as *specificity*. While substantially correct, specificity has in some instances (see below) been misleadingly overstated in a way that fails to do justice to the more recent evidence for *plasticity*.

To retain a balanced account of the scientific evidence, we need to remember that more than half a century ago workers such as Kretch, Rosenzweig, and Bennett showed how the physical and social environments of animals can

3. Coakley, introduction, p. 10.
4. Coakley, introduction, p. 14.
5. W. S. Brown, "The Brain, Religion, and Baseball: Comments on the Potential for a Neurology of Religion and Religious Experience," in *Where God and Science Meet: How Brain and Evolutionary Studies Alter Our Understanding of Religion*, vol. 2: *The Neurology of Religious Experience*, ed. P. McNamara (Westport, CT: Praeger, 2006), 242.
6. Brown, "Brain, Religion, and Baseball," 242.

shape and mold their brains as they grow to adulthood.[7] Similar research, using increasingly sophisticated methods, has brought recent results, such as those by Matthews and others, demonstrating the long-term effects of the early environment on adult behavior in the form of quite specific changes in the biochemistry of the brain and in concentrations of different neurotransmitters.[8] More recently, advances in the development of brain-scanning techniques have led to a fresh awareness of how cognitive processes and the social as well as the physical environment can "mold" or "sculpt" the brain (see for example Ian Robertson's 1999 book *Mind Sculpture*).[9] Studies such as these, reviewed by Robertson, together give new prominence to the actual and potential importance of so-called top-down processes.

The increasing demonstration of the intimate links between cognitive processes and brain processes may give clues to the possible neurobiological effects of beliefs and expectations. Advances in understanding the possible power of top-down effects have been so fast that what ten years ago leading researchers such as Grabowski and Damasio could see as "only a dream" has already been partially realized by researches such as those by O'Craven and Kanwisher and others, which are described later in this chapter.[10]

What has all this to do with the spiritual dimensions of healing? In brief, we assume that spirituality involves experience, belief, and action: experience in terms of our awareness of the transcendent, beliefs in terms of what we believe about God, ourselves, and the world in which we live, and action in terms of how we live our lives. The evidence that follows will highlight the intimate interdependence between brain processes, cognitive processes, and behavior and is relevant to understanding how those aspects of spirituality that mobilize and depend upon cognitive processes are not free-floating but firmly *embodied*. Such embodied beliefs and expectations are major factors in understanding some of the spiritual dimensions of healing. At the same time, we shall argue for the

7. M. R. Rosenzweig, D. Kretch, and E. L. Bennett, "Brain Chemistry and Adaptive Behavior," in *Biological and Biochemical Bases of Behavior*, ed. H. H. Harlow and C. N. Woolsey (Madison: University of Wisconsin Press, 1958), 367–400.

8. K. J. Matthews, J. W. Dalley, C. Matthews, Tung Hu Tsai, and T. W. Robbins, "Periodic Maternal Separation of Neonatal Rats Produces Region and Gender-Specific Effects on Biogenic Amine Content in Post-Mortem Adult Brain," *Synapse* 40 (2001): 1–10.

9. Ian Robertson, *Mind Sculpture* (New York: Bantam, 1999).

10. T. J. Grabowski and A. R. Damasio, "Improving Functional Imaging Techniques: The Dream of a Single Image for a Single Mental Event," *Proceedings of the National Academy of Sciences* 93 (1996): 14302–3; and K. M. O'Craven and N. Kanwisher, "Mental Imagery of Faces and Places Activates Corresponding Stimulus-Specific Brain Regions," *Journal of Cognitive Neuroscience* 12 (2000): 1013–23.

need to recognize that cognitive processes such as beliefs and expectations are frequently held within social contexts, and that reminds us that spirituality is also firmly *embedded*. Aspects of this *embeddedness* are clearly illustrated by Beverly Gaventa in chapter 1 in this volume as she discusses biblical perspectives on spiritual healing.

A Brief Historical Perspective

Human curiosity about the mind and how it is related to the body and, more specifically, to the brain has left a rich legacy of possible models from Plato and Aristotle, through Galen and Nemesius, to Descartes. Two millennia ago, Galen, surgeon to the gladiators, noted how selective brain damage incurred in combat resulted in differing sensory and motor deficits. It has, however, been only in the past two centuries that sustained attempts have been made to investigate mind-brain relations systematically. For the first hundred years of the past two centuries, the emphasis was largely on observing how mental life and behavior changed when accidental damage occurred to the human brain. Such accidental injury included the effects of strokes and disease as well as more traumatic head injuries. During the same period, attempts were made by the use of carefully designed animal experiments to undertake more controlled observations of the effects of localized brain damage on behavior. Thus, the effects of lesions on learning, seeing, remembering, and movement were studied. This type of approach is often labeled as "bottom-up." Martha Farah suggested that "a bottom-up approach begins with the most elementary levels of description believing that it will be impossible to understand higher levels of organization if one does not know precisely what is being organized."[11] Alternatively, Sarter and others suggest that "bottom-up approaches tend to be found in the lower levels of description in the basic neurosciences" and that, in using these approaches, "the attempt is made to understand the neural bases of cognitive phenomena by manipulating neural events."[12]

Another major approach to the understanding of mind-brain relations has been described as the "top-down" approach. In her review, Farah defined top-down approaches as the research strategy "according to which the most efficient

11. M. J. Farah, "Neuropsychological Inference with an Interactive Brain: A Critique of the 'Locality' Assumption," *Behavioral and Brain Sciences* 17 (1994): 44.

12. M. Sarter, G. G. Berntson, and J. T. Cacioppo, "Brain Imaging and Cognitive Neuroscience," *American Psychologist* 51, no. 1 (January 1996): 14.

way to understand the nervous system is by successive stages of analysis of systems of higher levels of description in terms of lower levels of description. It is argued that our understanding of lower levels will be facilitated if we know what high-level function they serve."[13] Sarter suggests that in top-down approaches, "the aim is to understand the neural bases of cognitive phenomena by manipulating cognitive events."[14]

For our present purposes, it is important to recognize that within cognitive and behavioral neuroscience, there is an ongoing discussion about how best to define top-down and bottom-up approaches. Top-down approaches are clearly of more relevance when considering spiritual dimensions of healing, since they may properly be extended to include cognitive events, such as changes in focus of attention, in beliefs, in anticipations, and in expectations. The evidence currently available supports the view that changes in such cognitive events appear to be paralleled by selective changes in brain activity. Howard Fields's chapter gives detailed support for this in his account of placebo effects. It is in this context that the very rapid developments and increasing sophistication of brain imaging techniques have given a new momentum to major research in this field.

The relevance of one of the conclusions of Sarter and others, however, remains important in any wider discussions of top-down effects and in any possible extrapolations such as we are engaged in here. In the decade since their paper appeared, the sophistication of brain-imaging methods has begun to make possible more precise localization of function, something that was lacking in many of the earlier studies. Nevertheless, there remains an ongoing debate about the "fundamental limitations in the strength of the inferences produced from experimental approaches aimed solely at the demonstration of $P(\Phi/\Psi)$," which is to say that when a change occurs in cognition, a change also occurs selectively in brain activation. Sarter and colleagues' more optimistic conclusion also remains relevant: "the integration of methods from bottom-up and top-down approaches provides a means of circumventing some of the thornier interpretive problems of either approach alone and thereby permits strong inferences in cognitive neuroscience."[15]

In the context of our considerations of the spiritual dimensions of healing, we shall see that, on the one hand, bottom-up approaches give special insights into understanding how changes in the neural structures of the brain, such as those occurring in Alzheimer's disease, manifest themselves in the subjective

---

13. Farah, "Neuropsychological Inference," 60.
14. Sarter, Berntson, and Cacioppo, "Brain Imaging and Cognitive Neuroscience," 14.
15. Sarter, Berntson, and Cacioppo, "Brain Imaging and Cognitive Neuroscience," 18–19.

awareness and the objective expression of the religious life, and, on the other hand, how top-down effects might give clues to how beliefs and expectations may operate in phenomena such as the placebo effect. Thus, as the progressive changes in the brains of Alzheimer's patients may manifest themselves in changes in their thoughts and beliefs, including religious ones, so the expectations manipulated in some studies of placebo effects manifest themselves in the individuals' biological substrates, including physical symptoms. In other words, the spiritual dimensions of our lives are both firmly *embodied* so that they do not remain immune to the effects of changes in brain and *embedded* so that they may sculpt our brains and be efficacious in healing.

Bottom-Up Approaches to the Study of Mind-Brain Links

In our brief look at the relevant background to understanding the current scene, it was noted that historically bottom-up methods dominated for a century and a half. Typical experimental procedures were to make changes in selective neural or biochemical substrates of the brain and then observe how behavior or cognitive capacities changed as a result. Soon it was not even necessary to produce surgical lesions, since, following on the pioneering work of Hubel and Wiesel, there was a rapid expansion in methods that depended upon implanting very small electrodes in columns of cells in the brain.[16] Researchers then monitored the activity in those cells, as the subjects, usually animals, were presented with a variety of sensory stimuli.

An example from the laboratories where I worked for three decades will help to illustrate the remarkable *specificity* of some aspects of neural processing. Thirty years ago, David Perrett and his colleagues at St. Andrews used single-cell recording techniques to map regions in monkey brains that responded selectively to the sight of human faces.[17] Every new study seemed to tighten the links between what the monkey was seeing and how the cells of the brain were

16. D. H. Hubel and T. N. Wiesel, "Receptive Fields of Single Neurones in the Cat's Striate Cortex," *Journal of Physiology* 148 (1959): 574–91.

17. See, for example, D. I. Perrett, P. A. J. Smith, D. D. Potter, A. J. Mistlin, A. S. Head, A. D. Milner, and M. A. Jeeves, "Neurons Responsive to Faces in the Temporal Cortex: Studies of Functional Organisation, Sensitivity to Identity and Relation to Perception," *Human Neurobiology* 3 (1984): 197–208; D. I. Perrett, J. K. Hietanen, M. W. Oram, and P. J. Benson, "Organization and Functions of Cells Responsive to Faces in the Temporal Cortex," *Philosophical Transactions of the Royal Biological Society* 335 (1992): 23–30; and D. I. Perrett, M. W. Oram, and E. Wachsmuth, "Understanding Minds and Expression from Facial Signals: Stud-

responding. There was a remarkable specificity in the cells' responses to facial stimuli. Among other things, Perrett found, for example, that changing the view of a face in its horizontal orientation from side profile to full face and back had a dramatic effect on the level of activity of face-responsive neurons. All of this suggested to Perrett that one of the key functions of these neurons may be to determine the direction of another's gaze. He proposed that the information provided by the eyes, the face, and the body was selectively processed by different columns of neurons, all part of a processing hierarchy for attention direction or social attention. Other researchers demonstrated that this was a part of a larger system.

With the advent of the so-called cognitive revolution (which was in part a reaction against behaviorism and, in part, reflected rapid developments by experimental psychologists of new methods to study mental events), new efforts were made to study how psychological processes were physically embodied in the brain. Research efforts by psychologists focused on memory, attention, and perception. It was not long before researchers such as Tulving could present a taxonomy that divided memory into working, or short-term, memory and long-term memory.[18] The latter was further subdivided into explicit and implicit long-term memory. Explicit long-term memory was further subdivided into episodic memory (for events) and semantic memory (for facts). Implicit long-term memory was divided into procedural and conceptual representational memory. Experimental psychologists devised ingenious techniques for studying these different sorts of memory empirically. Once this fractionation of cognitive processes had taken place, it led to a search for possible specific neural mechanisms upon which each of these forms of memory were dependent for their normal functioning. Such neural systems could be localized or widely spread throughout the brain.

Links between brain and mind are not confined to perception and cognition but also include the understanding of differences in human personality and behavior. Reports of such changes have appeared in the clinical literature from time to time and have a long and checkered history. Most who tell the story start with the account of how the railroad foreman Phineas Gage, working on the New England railroad, accidentally suffered damage to the frontal part of his brain and thereafter was a changed person. A dramatic example of a simi-

---

ied at the Brain Cell Level," *IEEE International Workshop on Robot and Human Communication* (1993): 3–12.

18. E. Tulving, *Elements of Episodic Memory* (Oxford: Clarendon, 1983).

lar change was reported recently by Burns and Swerdlow.[19] It described how a schoolteacher had begun collecting sex magazines and visiting pornographic websites and focusing his attention on images of children and adolescents. This was something that, according to him, he simply could not stop himself doing. He was arrested for child molestation, convicted, and underwent a rehabilitation program that was unsuccessful. The day before his final sentencing, he went voluntarily to the hospital emergency department complaining of a severe headache. He was distraught and contemplating suicide and was aware that he could not control his impulses — so much so that he propositioned the nurses in the hospital. An MRI scan of his brain revealed a large tumor pressing on his right frontal lobe. The surgeons removed it, and the lewd behavior and pedophilia faded away. Sadly, a year afterward he began to manifest pedophilia afresh. New MRI scans showed that the tumor was beginning to regrow. It was removed, and once again his urges subsided. This case, not surprisingly, received wide publicity and comment. One thing, however, is clear: it demonstrated the remarkably tight links between what is happening in the brain and how we behave.

Evidence about the remarkable *specificity* of localization of functions within the brain can lead to a serious failure to recognize the *plasticity* of the developing brain. Such an overemphasis is at times present in the work of the widely read author Steven Pinker.[20] He draws his evidence mainly from adult neuropsychological data and from genetic disorders involving language. However, other leading workers in the field, such as Karmiloff-Smith, have pointed out that in some instances, Pinker's interpretation of the data is flawed.[21] She notes that it is based on a static model of the human brain that ignores the complexities of gene expression and the dynamics of postnatal development (for more details see, for example, Michael Rutter).[22] The citation for Professor Karmiloff-Smith's award of the 2004 Latsis Prize by the European Science Foundation aptly sums up the importance of her corrective remarks. It observed that "Her research aimed to show that the brain is neither hardwired nor a blank slate, but that both genes and environment interact in complex ways and that the actual pro-

19. See J. M. Burns and R. H. Swerdlow, "Right Orbitofrontal Tumor with Pedophilia Symptoms and Constructional Apraxia Sign," *Archives of Neurology* 60, no. 3 (March 2003): 437–40.

20. Steven Pinker, *Words and Rules: The Ingredients of Language* (London: Wiedenfeld and Nicholson, 1999).

21. A. Karmiloff-Smith, "Elementary, My Dear Watson, the Clue Is in the Genes. Or Is It?," *Psychologist* 15, no. 12 (2002): 608–11.

22. M. Rutter, *Genes and Behaviour: Nature-Nurture Interplay Explained* (London: Blackwell, 2006).

cess of post-natal development plays a crucial role in this dynamic interaction," further adding, "this highlights the fact that the adult neuropsychological model is inappropriate for explaining developmental disorders."[23]

A similar point — in this context, the effects of *both* built-in genetic factors *and* early experience — has been made in a review paper by Nancy Kanwisher and Galit Yovel.[24] They adduce a large body of evidence for the specificity of neural mechanisms for face perception in the Fusiform Face Area. They argue that in the ongoing debate about the "extent to which the mind/brain is composed of a) special-purpose ('domain-specific') mechanisms, each dedicated to processing a specific kind of information (e.g. faces, according to the Face Specificity Hypothesis), versus b) general-purpose ('domain-general') mechanisms, each capable of operating on any kind of information." Furthermore, their work "supports the Face Specificity Hypothesis and argues against its domain-general alternatives." At the same time, they note that "evidence that very early experience is also crucial in the development of normal adult face recognition comes from studies of individuals born with dense bilateral cataracts." They conclude, "In sum, substantial evidence indicates important roles for both genetic factors and specific early experience, in the construction of the Fusiform Face Area" (the FFA is the face specific processing region of the brain).

Clearly, there is a remarkable specificity in the neural mechanisms for some of our most important perceptual and cognitive functions in social interactions and for daily living. At the same time, all of this further underlines that with specificity, there is also *plasticity*. As the example in the next section documents, specific dedicated brain regions change as a result of specific experiences. Recognizing the key importance of psychological processes and the evidence for *plasticity*, we turn now to consider the special relevance of top-down effects as we reflect on the spiritual dimensions of healing.

Top-Down Approaches to the Study of Mind-Brain Links

As the cognitive revolution has spread, ever more sophisticated brain imaging techniques have also been concurrently developed. Imaging research points to the importance of top-down effects, referring to changes in cognition being

---

23. Latsis Prize citation in Karmiloff-Smith, "Elementary, My Dear Watson," 611.

24. Nancy Kanwisher and Galit Yovel, "The Fusiform Face Area: A Cortical Region Specialized for the Perception of Faces," *Philosophical Transactions of the Royal Society* 361, no. 1476 (2006): 2109–28.

paralleled by localized changes in the brain. Two striking examples of top-down effects must suffice to illustrate their potency.

Maguire and his colleagues noted that licensed London taxi drivers are renowned for their extensive and detailed navigation experience and skills.[25] They collected structural MRIs of the brains of a group of taxi drivers and matched controls and discovered that, as a result of two years of intensive training in navigation, the anterior hippocampi of the taxi drivers were significantly larger. Moreover, the volume of grey matter in the right hippocampus correlated significantly with the amount of time spent as a taxi driver. The researchers concluded, "it seems that there is a capacity for local plastic changes in the structure of the healthy adult human brain in response to environmental demands."[26]

The second example is a study by O'Craven and Kanwisher (whose work on specificity was described above) that beautifully illustrates how the mind can selectively mobilize specific brain systems.[27] They asked volunteers to look at pictures of faces or houses or to imagine these pictures. They demonstrated how imagining faces or houses selectively activated the same areas of the brain as when the subjects were seeing the pictures of houses or faces. Specifically, seeing or thinking about faces activated the fusiform face area, while seeing or thinking about houses activated the parahippocampal place area. The experimenters in effect showed that they could actually "read the minds" of their subjects by observing their brain activity. They could tell whether the subjects were thinking about faces or houses by measuring activity in respective brain areas.

Once again, however, and lest we get carried away by an overemphasis on specificity, there comes a timely reminder in a report in the journal *NeuroReport*, the results of which underline the importance of recognizing *plasticity*.[28] The researchers studied a group of eighteen- to twenty-seven-year-olds and compared them with an equal number of sixty-one- to eighty-year-olds. They were given the task of remembering three images of houses or three images of faces and were then asked to decide whether another image was from the original set. Using functional magnetic resonance imaging (fMRI) techniques, the researchers tracked the neural changes while these tasks were being done. What they discovered was that the older adults showed decreased specialization in the

25. E. A. Maguire, D. G. Gadian, I. S. Johnsrude, C. D. Good, J. Ashburner, R. S. J. Frackopwiak, and C. Frith, "Navigation-Related Structural Change in the Hippocampi of Taxi Drivers," *Proceedings of the National Academy of Sciences* 97, no. 8 (2000): 4398–4403.

26. Maguire et al., "Navigation-Related Structural Change," 4398.

27. O'Craven and Kanwisher, "Mental Imagery of Faces and Places," 1013–23.

28. D. Payer, B. Sutton, A. Hebrank, and D. Park, "Decreased Specialization in Old Adults on a Working Memory Task," *NeuroReport* 17, no. 5 (April 3, 2006): 493–97.

two brain areas studied by O'Craven and Kanwisher when they were compared with the younger adults. They also found more activity in the older adults in the frontal cortex and suggested that this activity was in part compensation for less differentiation in the visual cortex at the back of the brain. The researchers noted, "This underscores the importance of taking into account the connected and networked nature of the brain and its function in understanding human neural ageing."[29] Thus, the role of developmental processes is important in later as well as early development.

A Balanced View

The picture emerging from the science briefly reviewed points to the intimate relationships between mind, brain, and behavior. We described some of these as bottom-up and some as top-down, in a particular sense outlined at the beginning of this chapter. There is now an emerging consensus about how to portray these intimate relationships. The neurologist Antonio Damasio wrote that "the distinction between diseases of brain and mind and between neurological problems and psychological/psychiatric ones, is an unfortunate cultural inheritance that permeates society and medicine. It reflects a basic ignorance of the relation between brain and mind."[30] A similar view was expressed by Robert Kendall, a past president of the Royal College of Psychiatrists in Britain. He wrote, "not only is the distinction between mental and physical ill founded and incompatible with contemporary understanding of disease, it is also damaging for the long-term interests of patients themselves."[31]

The relevance of this emerging consensus of views for our discussions of the spiritual dimensions of healing is that it emphasizes that our mental processes are not free-floating somewhere out in space but are firmly *embodied* in our physical makeup. At the same time, it prompts us to remember that the researches of cognitive scientists presented in terms of psychological processes will not vanish and are not explained away as we begin to understand something about how such processes are dependent upon the normal functioning of the human brain. There is so much yet to be discovered by cognitive scientists about, for example, the different types of memory, and only then can we ask sensible questions about how each of these is embodied in the brain.

29. Payer et al., "Decreased Specialization," 497.
30. A. Damasio, *Descartes' Error* (New York: Putnam, 1994), 40.
→ 31. R. E. Kendall, "The Distinction between Mental and Physical Illness," *British Journal of Psychiatry* 178 (2001): 490.

We noted earlier the advice of Sarter and colleagues that an effective strategy in trying to ensure that any inferences we make about the relations between psychological processes and their neural substrates is to remember that "the integration of methods and data from bottom-up and top-down approaches provides a means of circumventing some of the thornier interpretative problems of either approach alone and thereby permits strong inferences in cognitive neuroscience."[32] In this way, we can simultaneously remember that cognitive processes are embodied within the brain and sculpt the brain. It is clear that while there is a remarkable *specificity* about how some of our most fundamental perceptual and cognitive processes are embodied in our brains, there is also striking evidence of how cognition and behavior sculpt our brains, demonstrating equally remarkable *plasticity*.

Mind and Brain, Body and Soul: Relationships of Irreducible, Intrinsic, Interdependence?

Some discussions of human nature tend quickly to focus upon the relative claims of dualism and monism. When this happens, monistic views are often made synonymous with physicalism and are further portrayed as necessarily materialist and reductionist. In short, a great deal of philosophic baggage invariably gets attached to the terms *monism*, *dualism*, and *physicalism*. Can this be avoided in a way that underlines the *unity* of the person while at the same time recognizing the need for a *duality* of accounts, if we are to do full justice to the way the world is?

Studies by neuropsychologists such as those described above underlined the dependence of the mental aspects of our life on their physical embodiments in the brain and the body. Such evidence indicated the remarkable *interdependence* between what is happening in the physical substrates, in terms of brain and body mechanisms, and what is happening in terms of mental abilities and individual and social behavior. While interdependence is not denied by Cartesian dualists, the nature of the interdependence increasingly uncovered by scientific research, we believe, makes a substance dualism harder to maintain without tortuous and convoluted reasoning. The burgeoning field of psycho-neuro-immunology also produces example after example of the way in which observed changes in the social situation and mental life are reflected in observable changes in cerebral and endocrine processes.

It is one thing to demonstrate the intimate interrelationship between what is happening at the conscious mental level and what is happening at the level

32. Sarter, Berntson, and Cacioppo, "Brain Imaging and Cognitive Neuroscience," 13.

of the brain and the body. But the unanswered question is how can we most accurately characterize this intimate relationship without making claims or assumptions about what we know regarding the relationship between the two, which have not yet been demonstrated? What is clear is that there is a remarkable *interdependence* between what is occurring at the cognitive level and what is occurring at the physical level. We could perhaps describe this as a relationship of *intrinsic interdependence*, using the word *intrinsic* to mean that, as far as we can see, it describes the way the world is in this regard. Could we perhaps go further than this and say that on our present knowledge it is an *irreducible intrinsic interdependence*, by this meaning that *we cannot reduce the mental to the physical any more than we can reduce the physical to the mental? In this sense, there is an important duality to be recognized, but it is a duality without dualism.*

Any reference to dualism will for many readers make immediate links with centuries of debates by theologians and philosophers about the body and the soul and how these are related. However, it is important to remember that for anyone interested in the relevance of what the Hebrew and Christian Scriptures have to say on this topic, we need to remember that fine philosophical distinctions are not the business of the biblical authors. For example, Joel Green has remarked,

> The Bible's witness to the nature of human life is at once naïve and profound. It is naïve, not in the sense of gullibility or primitiveness, but because it has not worked out, in what we may regard as a philosophically satisfying way, the nature of physical existence in life, death, and afterlife. It is profound in its presentation of the human person fundamentally in relational terms, and its assessment of the human being as genuinely human and alive only within the family of humans brought into being by Yahweh and in relation to the God who gives life-giving breath.[33]

People sometimes liken this *irreducible intrinsic interdependence* that manifests *duality without dualism* to the interdependence of computer software and computer hardware. Even here, however, there are traps for the unwary. All too easily, analogies of the relationship between mental events and physical events, or software and hardware, are smuggled in as if they were explanations.

Some time ago the late Professor Donald MacKay suggested that it was silly to pit the mental and physical levels of description against one another; rather,

33. J. B. Green, "Eschatology and the Nature of Humans: A Reconsideration of Pertinent Biblical Evidence," *Science and Christian Belief* 14 (2002): 38.

they should be seen as harmoniously complementary.[34] The mental at the conscious level is spelling out the personal significance (echoes of Coakley's "religious meaning systems"?) of a unitary situation. The physical is dealing with another aspect of it, the so-called brain story. Donald MacKay was keen, when using the computer analogy, to emphasize that between the descriptions at the software and hardware level, there is a correlation, but this is not a translation. The example he liked to use was that if we have a mathematical equation that has two roots and it is embodied in a computer, then the facts about the equation are not facts about the computer, except, as he put it, in a "Pickwickian" sense. He wrote, "computers don't have roots."[35] And yet if the computer is solving the equation, there is a direct physical correlate for the statement "the equation has two roots," and any engineer can tell you what it is. But no one is suggesting that if you look hard enough you can find roots in the computer.

Eminent neuroscientist and Nobel Laureate Roger Sperry went to considerable lengths, in his opposition to a climate of dominant behaviorism in American psychology at that time, to emphasize the importance of the cognitive aspects of behavior with his reference to top-down effects.[36] Indeed, to make his point, at times, he went so far as to refer to mental activity as "pushing and hauling" the activity of the brain. We are suggesting that if one is embodied in the other, then the interdependence is even closer than "pushing and hauling." Sperry's words can be read as implying that the mental manipulates the physical, and that can too easily be read as giving priority to the mental, something Sperry did not wish to do. Rather, what we are anxious to affirm, as was MacKay, is that the mental activity is efficacious in determining the activity of the brain. That does not mean that you spend your time trying to find elements in the physics of the computer "sensitive" to influences from the hypothetical mathematical world. Hence, between the mental and the physical, there is an *irreducible* (in the sense that to get rid of either is to tell less than the whole story), *intrinsic* (in the sense that it is part of the way the world is) *interdependence* (the mental and physical are correlated and complementary), reflecting *duality but not dualism* of substance. From the point of view of the logic of the metaphysics of Western language-usage, as far as people are concerned, the prime ontological term is *person*, as the individual subject of whom we assert two types of predicates, men-

34. See D. M. MacKay, *Behind the Eye* (Oxford: Blackwell, 1991), 60.

35. MacKay, *Behind the Eye*, 60.

36. Roger Sperry, "Forebrain Commissurotomy and Conscious Awareness," in *Brain Circuits and Functions of the Mind: Essays in Honor of Roger W. Sperry*, ed. Colwyn W. Trevarthen (Cambridge: Cambridge University Press, 1990), 382–85.

tal and physical. There is thus a duality, but not dualism: the ontological reality of *person* is primary and is neither mental nor physical.

Embodied Spirituality

The possibility, let alone the probability, of a volume being written on the neurology of religion would have seemed most unlikely three decades ago. The reality is that advance notice has already been given of just such a forthcoming volume. In an earlier section, I referred to spirituality as, in part, awareness of the transcendental, as well as the holding of certain beliefs. The link between spirituality and brain processes has a long well-documented history — for example, in the close association between certain forms of epilepsy and exceptional religiosity.

As in the case of the top-down studies described above, it has been the rapid sophistication in brain-imaging techniques applied to the study of religious behavior that has given rise to the very rapid increase in this field, sometimes described as neurotheology and other times as theoneurology. There are potential benefits from good research in neurotheology, such as giving a fresh understanding of the etiology of some bizarre manifestations of religiosity with the possibility of bringing relief through tailored and targeted psychotropic drugs. In the context of this current volume on spiritual healing — or, as more narrowly conceived in this chapter, on the spiritual dimensions of healing — the importance and the relevance of these developments is that they point to the accumulating evidence supporting a view that spirituality is firmly embodied in our biological makeup.

In the meantime, exaggerated claims and overinterpretation of some of the findings from neurotheology call for the kind of sober assessments given by Jerome Groopman and Mario Beauregard. Groopman, a distinguished Jewish physician, wrote, "Why do we have this strange attempt, clothed in the rubric of 'neurotheology,' to objectify faith with the bells and whistles of technology?," later adding, "Man is a proper subject for study in the world of science . . . God is not."[37] Similar views were echoed by Mario Beauregard, who works in the departments of radiology and psychology at the University of Montreal and who was reported by Christopher Stawski as saying, "Obviously, the external reality of God can be neither confirmed nor disconfirmed by delineating neural correlates of religious/spiritual/mystical experiences. In other words, the neu-

---

37. J. Groopman, "God on the Brain," *New Yorker*, September 17, 2001, 168.

roscientific study of what happens to the brain during these experiences does not tell us anything new about God."[38]

Any belief that our spirituality is securely protected within an immaterial part of us labeled the soul is most obviously challenged by the common experience of carers of loved ones who have developed Alzheimer's disease. Some of these deeply religious people have suffered agonizing distress as they have subjectively witnessed the fragmentation of some of the most precious aspects of their religious life and experience. Such distress has been equally agonizing to their loved ones and carers.

Glenn Weaver, who has developed a large research program into the changes in spirituality in Alzheimer's patients, has listed some of the experiences of self-identity changes frequently linked to the changes in these individuals' experiences of spiritual meanings and faith.[39] The consequences to the individual of the development of Alzheimer's dementia may vary widely. For example, Weaver describes in detail the experiences of the Rev. Robert Davis, a Presbyterian minister, diagnosed with Alzheimer's dementia when he was fifty-three and at the height of his ministerial career. With the help of his wife, he wrote a remarkable account of his spiritual experiences well into the middle stages of the disease. How his progressive brain disease affected his spirituality is graphically illustrated in his own words. He wrote:

> My spiritual life was miserable. I could not read the Bible. I could not pray as I wanted to because my emotions were dead and cut off. There was no feedback from God the Holy Spirit. My mind could not rest and grow calm but raced relentlessly thinking dreadful thoughts of despair. . . . I can no longer be spiritually fed by sermons. I can get the first point of the sermon and then am lost. The rest of it sends my mind whirling in a jumble of twisted unconnected ideas. Coughing, headache and great discomfort have attended my attempts to be fed in all the ways I am accustomed to, meeting God through his Word. . . . My mind also raced about, grasping for the comfort of the Savior whom I knew and loved and the emotional peace that He could give me, but finding nothing. I concluded that the only reason for such darkness must be spiritual. Unnamed guilt filled me. Yet the only guilt I could put a

---

38. C. Stawski and M. Beauregard, "Spiritual Transformation Q and A: Mario Beauregard," *Global Spiral* 4, no. 3 (March 1, 2004): 249.

39. G. Weaver, "Embodied Spirituality: Experiences of Identity and Spiritual Suffering among Persons with Alzheimer's Dementia," in *From Cells to Souls — and Beyond*, ed. Malcolm Jeeves (Grand Rapids: Eerdmans, 2004), 77–101.

name on was failure to read my Bible. But I could not read, and would God condemn me for this? I could only lie there and cry "Oh God, why? why?"[40]

Thus, while there is little doubt that spirituality is firmly embodied in our biological makeup, any wider discussion under headings such as "the neurology of religion" must be seen as no more than a convenient summary for what is in reality a neurology of the cognitive contributions to specific behaviors and experiences labeled by the individual as "religious," the latter resulting from personal beliefs and behaviors in social contexts. It is to these social contexts that we now turn as we consider the *embeddedness* of spirituality.

Embedded Spirituality

Except in very rare instances such as the lonely hermit, the spiritual dimensions to life and experience are lived out in community. In a word, as with all other aspects of our daily existence, our spirituality develops, is maintained, and manifests itself in community. It is fully embedded in our physical, cultural, and social environments. In the context of our discussions of the spiritual dimensions of healing, this brings to mind the substantial body of social-psychological research, extending over many decades, linking personal and group beliefs with well-being.

Reviewing the literature on the link between social support and health, David Myers points out that environments that support our need to belong also foster a stronger immune functioning.[41] He notes that social ties and positive sociability can even confer resistance to cold viruses, and how more than fifty studies reveal that social support calms the cardiovascular system, lowering blood pressure and stress hormones. Relevant to our present discussions of the spiritual dimensions of healing, it is noteworthy that throughout history, as Myers points out, the healing traditions — religion and medicine — have joined hands in caring for suffering humans. At times those hands belonged to the same person.

As medical science developed, healing and religion tended to diverge. No longer did people ask God to spare their children from smallpox — they took them to be vaccinated; rather than seeking a spiritual healer in the face of bacterial fever, they applied antibiotics. This trend to separate medicine and reli-

---

40. Weaver, "Embodied Spirituality," 89–90.
41. See D. Myers, *Psychology*, 8th ed. (New York: Worth, 2006), esp. ch. 14.

gion, however, has been reversed in a remarkable way in recent decades, particularly in North America, where religion and healing seem to be converging once again.

In his review, Myers notes that more than one thousand studies have now sought to correlate the so-called faith factor with health and healing. He cites as one of the most important of the studies the one described by Anne Harrington in her chapter in this volume — namely, the work by Kark and his colleagues who in 1996 compared the death rates of thirty-nine hundred Israelis living either in one of eleven religiously orthodox or in eleven matched nonreligious collective settlements-kibbutzim.[42] As Harrington notes, belonging to the religious collective appeared to be associated with a strong protective effect against ill health. How to understand these results will remain a matter of debate and further investigation for some years. It may be that the religious beliefs of the kibbutzim members resulted in a potentiation of the already acknowledged beneficial effects of social support of kibbutzim in coping with illness and disease. David Myers notes that researchers in this field speculate that even after taking note of variables such as gender, unhealthy behaviors, social ties, and preexisting health problems, there remain a third set of intervening variables that confer stress protection and enhanced well-being; they are associated with a coherent worldview, a sense of hope for the long-term future, feelings of ultimate acceptance, and the relaxed meditation of prayer or Sabbath observance. Each of these may be seen as part of the spiritual dimensions at work in some forms of healing.

Conclusion

We have seen how the results of research at the interface of psychology and neuroscience have underlined the intimate relationships between mind and brain. I have suggested that a helpful way to think about the relationship between the mental and physical aspects of our life is one of irreducible intrinsic interdependence that manifests duality without dualism.

While some of the research findings as reported in the media are dramatic, many unanswered questions remain about how properly to interpret them. It is also clear that this is very much a report of work "in progress." There is an ongoing lively debate among those at the cutting edge of the research, as well

42. J. D. Kark, S. Carmel, R. Sinnreich, N. Goldberger, and Y. Friedlander, "Psychosocial Factors among Members of Religious and Secular Kibbutzim," *Israel Journal of Medical Science* 32, nos. 3–4 (March–April 1996): 185–94.

as among philosophers, about how best to make sense of it all. There are no simple slick answers.

A salient feature of neuropsychological research over the past three decades has been the increasing recognition of the importance of so-called top-down effects. By the mid-1990s reports of top-down effects were appearing with increasing frequency in the literature. In 1994 Martha Farah produced a timely review of the use of the terms *top-down* and *bottom-up* and brought a necessary corrective to some of the looser usage of these terms.[43] In his chapter in this volume, Howard Fields gave an excellent example of how some of these top-down effects have been explored experimentally in the instance of placebo effects.[44] We have given examples from other areas of neuropsychology in this chapter, noting their relevance to our topic of spiritual healing. References by other contributors to this volume of the importance of beliefs, expectations, hopes, and anticipations of healing, whether by individuals or by groups, indicate the relevance of top-down effects for any discussion of the spiritual dimensions of healing. While our mental processes, beliefs, hopes, and expectations are firmly *embodied* in our biological makeup, notably our brains, they are also *embedded* within social contexts of shared beliefs, behaviors, and attitudes. These also have effects.

In her chapter on the biblical perspectives of spiritual healing, Beverly Gaventa writes, "Healing is integrally involved with community — whether that community be a small local gathering or the whole of Israel. Indeed, the community's role in the phenomenon of spiritual healing is far more extensive than might be imagined simply by noticing the presence of crowds as witnesses in the Gospel stories of Jesus's healing. In fact, the community is itself deeply implicated in the biblical phenomenon of spiritual healing."[45] She takes up this theme later when she writes, "In some instances, the community itself takes on the more active role, becoming the agent of healing," and later, "These diverse strands of the New Testament share the same audacious claim that spiritual healing is located within the believing community."[46] All of this, what we might describe as *embeddedness* in the horizontal dimension, is also to be read as we constantly remember that "healing has to do with God's will for human flourishing, with the reclamation of all of creation," as Gaventa reminds us with allusion to Romans 8. In other words, healing in Scripture is *horizontally embedded* within

43. Farah, "Neuropsychological Inference," 43–61.
44. Howard L. Fields, chapter 4, pp. 92–93.
45. Gaventa, chapter 1, p. 34.
46. Gaventa, chapter 1, p. 36.

the believing community and *vertically embedded* within the purposes of God's will for human flourishing — a God who, Christians believe, upholds all things at all times by the word of his power.

For our generation, so used to watching plays on our televisions, we may ask, might this provide a helpful way of thinking about the *horizontal* as well as the *vertical* dimensions of God's activity? In watching any play, we soon become aware of the relationships between the participants in the story and of how both their behavior individually and their social behavior may be influenced by the physical and social environment within which they live. We work out person-to-person causal relationships as well as between people and environmental, social, and physical events. At the same time, we know that the author of the whole play is, in a very real sense, generating, upholding, and controlling everything that we see on our screens. If we give our author the added privilege of being the owner of the transmitting station, then, in a real sense, the whole show that we observe can be fully attributed to his creative and sustaining activity. Is this one way we may begin to think about spiritual healing?

In light of the increasing likelihood that, with advances in our scientific understanding of human nature, we may be able, in due time, to provide natural explanations of unusual healings, do we need to reemphasize our Christian belief in a moment-by-moment Creator, an Upholding-God? Such a view, while fully recognizing that the spiritual dimensions of healing are both *embodied* and *embedded*, thankfully affirms that the whole show, all that we observe and are privileged to study about it, is concurrently a manifestation of the unchanging and steadfast love of a Creator God who upholds all things at all times, and not the product of an interventionist magician.[47]

---

47. For more expanded discussion on the topics discussed in this chapter, see Malcolm Jeeves, *Minds, Brains, Souls and Gods: A Conversation on Neuroscience, Psychology and Religion* (Downers Grove, IL: IVP Academic, 2013).

6

Prayer and Placebo in Scientific Research

Anne Harrington

In the last two chapters, we have looked at the insights of neuroscience and psychology on the topic of spiritual healing. We now turn to the issue of how the history of science should review this domain of discussion, and in particular how it should assess recent attempts to catch instances of spiritual healing in the web of scientific verification. But this immediately drives us back to fundamental issues, which cannot be gainsaid. So, once again, we ask the basic questions: How should we define spiritual healing? How should we think about its aims? How should we assess medical and scientific evidence of its effectiveness?

The most important point is that all of these questions are *normative*: that is, they already suppose an ability on our part to develop criteria for a best-practice approach to research and scholarship on spiritual healing. As an historian of science and medicine, however, I am disciplinarily biased to feel that we must be diagnostic before we can be prescriptive. Who is already out there defining spiritual healing, thinking about its aims, and deciding on norms for assessing evidence of its effectiveness? And what do we think about the job these other people are doing?

Recent efforts in the United States to study the effectiveness of intercessory prayer on the healing process — an intervention that I assume will be generally acknowledged as a spiritual-healing practice — offer themselves as one arena where we can attempt to be a bit diagnostic before we become prescriptive. Moreover, the prominence of such studies — the fact that many people have perceived so much to be at stake in their outcomes — may make it a particularly appropriate case to examine in some detail.

Prayer Research and the Religion-Health Connection

In the United States, prayer studies first established themselves as a special sub-field of a larger research effort to investigate the health benefits of religious practice and belief more generally. One of the things I want to argue is that this fact is critical for understanding, at least in part, why they have been designed in the way that they have. Before turning to the prayer studies themselves, let us therefore briefly review the research agenda of the larger territory studies designed to assess the health benefits of religion more generally, of which efforts to assess the efficacy of prayer are — for better or worse — a part.

The first and perhaps most straightforward item on that agenda is concerned with the possibility that church attendance is good for your health. The origins of this claim lie in epidemiological work that began in the late 1960s. This was a time of great medical interest in identifying the lifestyle and environmental factors that were contributing to the rising incidence of heart disease, especially in the United States. Out of this work, social isolation emerged as a potentially important factor. Some work suggested, for example, that living in traditional close-knit communities protects against heart disease and, possibly, other common forms of morbidity and mortality. Other studies indicated that more isolated people within a community tend to be sicker and to die earlier than those who are more socially embedded.[1]

The epidemiologists who first undertook this sort of work did not start out intending to investigate the possibility that religion is good medicine. From the beginning, however, membership in a religious community was included as one independent variable among many others that might act as measures of social embeddedness, and it soon became clear that it was a particularly important one. Various kinds of work began to suggest that church attendance was strongly correlated with a reduced likelihood of suffering from any number of health problems, especially in old age. Some studies even suggested that going to church was correlated with extended lifespan.[2]

What might be the reason for this? The most common answer in the liter-

---

1. Some classic reference points in this literature include L. F. Berkman and S. L. Syme, "Social Networks, Host Resistance and Mortality: A Nine Year Follow-Up Study of Alameda County Residents," *American Journal of Epidemiology* 109 (1979): 186–204; J. G. Bruhn and S. Wolf, *The Roseto Story* (Norman: University of Oklahoma Press, 1979); S. Wolf, "Predictors of Myocardial Infarction over a Span of 30 Years in Roseto, Pennsylvania," *Integrative Physiological and Behavioral Science* 27, no. 3 (1992): 246–57; J. S. House, K. R. Landis, and D. Umberson, "Social Relationships and Health," *Science* 241, no. 4865 (1988): 540–45.

2. See, for example, W. J. Strawbridge, R. D. Cohen, and G. A. Kaplan, "Frequent Atten-

ature has been that churches (and, by extension, synagogues and mosques) are good for your health because they provide exceptionally good social support. Religious communities tend to look after their members, they tend to frown on unhealthy behaviors like excess alcohol and drugs, and — in being publicly concerned about each other's health — they might even tend to create a culture in which individuals seek medical assistance earlier than they otherwise might have.

That said, not everyone has been satisfied that reducing churchgoing to social support was an adequate explanation for the data. For example, in 1996, the Israeli epidemiologist Jeremy Kark compared mortality rates in eleven secular and eleven matched religious kibbutzim between 1970 and 1985 and found that mortality in the secular kibbutzim was twice that of mortality in the religious kibbutzim. At the same time, he and his colleagues insisted, *"there was no difference in social support or frequency of social contact between religious and secular kibbutzim."*[3]

Findings like these led some to suggest that social support is an inadequate explanation for the data linking church attendance to improvement on various health measures. What kind of explanation, then, might be more adequate? Two sorts are discernible in the literature. The first of these focuses on the putative stress-reducing effects of the various kinds of spiritual practices that are generally part of a committed faith: prayer, meditation, ritual chanting, and so on.[4] The second focuses on the ways in which strong faith might be able to "turn on" endogenous physiological healing processes and grounds its claims in indirect evidence drawn from new kinds of research on the placebo effect. After being derided or ignored for years, the placebo effect — the tendency for patients' *belief* in the efficacy of a medication to make them feel better — has been rehabilitated in our own time as a phenomenon that we now believe is capable

dance at Religious Services and Mortality over 28 Years," *American Journal of Public Health* 87 (1997): 957–61.

3. J. D. Kark, S. Carmel, R. Sinnreich, N. Goldberger, Y. Friedlander, "Psychosocial Factors among Members of Religious and Secular Kibbutzim," *Israeli Journal of Medical Science* 32, nos. 3–4 (March–April 1996): 185–94.

4. See, for example, the influential work of Herbert Benson on these issues: R. K. Wallace, H. Benson, and A. F. Wilson, "A Wakeful Hypometabolic State," *American Journal of Physiology* 221 (1971): 795–99; R. K. Wallace and H. Benson, "The Physiology of Meditation," *Scientific American* 226, no. 2 (1972): 84–90; J. F. Beary and H. Benson, "A Simple Physiologic Technique Which Elicits the Hypometabolic Changes of the Relaxation Response," *Psychosomatic Medicine* 36 (1974): 115–20; Benson's best-selling book (with Marion Z. Klipper) popularizing his technique and its health-promoting effects was *The Relaxation Response* (New York: Morrow, 1975).

of producing real — physiologically measurable — effects.[5] If a person's belief in medicine (and the biochemistry associated with such belief) can cause changes in his or her body, then why should not belief in a God who heals also be able to produce similar — or perhaps even *more* powerful — salubrious changes? Some have even suggested that we humans may have evolved with a strong tendency to expect healing from powerful entities (like gods or doctors) in part because of the physiological changes such expectations seem to trigger.[6]

The Placebo Effect and Spiritual Healing: A Closer Look

What relevance do these developments have for our concerns? A brief historical excursion may help clarify the issues. Of specific interest is the case of Lourdes in the late nineteenth century, not long after it was sanctioned as a pilgrimage site and healing shrine by the Catholic Church.[7] The church did indeed recognize Lourdes as a place where authentic spiritual healings might happen, but it did so in a way that it hoped would allow it to maintain its authority to pass judgment on people's experience and, in this way, to ensure that Lourdes did not spiral into a populist movement that it could not control.[8] One of the most important ways in which it did this was by establishing a medical bureau composed of physicians whose mandate was to decide which of the many claimed miracle healings at Lourdes were *in fact* "medically inexplicable," as judged from a range of objective criteria. (The question whether medically inexplicable healings were genuinely miraculous was a theological matter, and so final judgment on every case was to be left to the clerics.)

In making its judgments, the medical bureau was deeply influenced by recent research in secular French medicine into such phenomena as hysteria and hypnosis that collectively had led to a deep suspicion of the human mind, and especially of the minds of (often poor, often female) patients. It was generally understood that, unwittingly, the mind — influenced by "suggestion" and its

5. On the placebo effect, see, among others, A. Harrington, ed., *The Placebo Effect: An Interdisciplinary Exploration* (Cambridge: Harvard University Press, 1997).

6. Nicholas Humphrey, "Great Expectations: The Evolutionary Psychology of Faith-Healing and the Placebo Response," in *Proceedings of the 27th International Congress of Psychology*, ed. Lars Backman and Claes von Hofsten (New York: Psychology, 2000).

7. For a complementary account to the one given here, see Emma Anderson's contribution to this volume, chapter 2.

8. A good introduction to the history of Lourdes and the management of its miracles is Ruth Harris's *Lourdes: Body and Spirit in the Secular Age* (New York: Viking, 1999).

own "imagination" — often essentially fabricated experiences and even physical symptoms that nevertheless could not be taken at face value. The mind was a trickster, and the job of medicine was to learn its tricks so as not to be fooled by them.

At the same time, efforts to distinguish pseudomiracles wrought by suggestion's power from true miracles wrought by God were actually important in two ways to the medical bureau: the goal was not just to debunk and expose pseudohealings but also to call attention to the apparent inability of the new French ideas about the power of the mind (the "power of suggestion") to account for a lot of what was going on at Lourdes. Could suggestion, for example, account for the disappearance of tumors in patients who had taken the waters? In the words of one of the clerics at the time:

> The most learned and daring of the suggestionists of the present day, Bernheim, a Jew, head of the famous school of Nancy . . . answers in the negative. . . . Therefore curative suggestion is no explanation. It is not suggestion that operates at Lourdes; the cause which cures acts differently and is infinitely more powerful. . . . As a matter of fact, no natural cause, known or unknown, is sufficient to account for the marvelous cures witnessed at the foot of the celebrated rock where the Virgin Immaculate deigned to appear. They can only be from the intervention of God.[9]

It is at this point, perhaps rather improbably, that two former rivals from the world of French hysteria and hypnosis research, Hippolyte Bernheim and Jean-Martin Charcot, found themselves united in mutual indignation. Both of them secularists to the core, with no love for the Catholic Church (Charcot was openly anticlerical, Bernheim a secular Jew), it was a grave affront to them both that clergy from the Catholic Church should misappropriate medical discussions of the time about the limits of suggestion's power in order to advance spurious supernaturalist arguments. In no sense were these men prepared to agree that, where suggestion let off, God began. On the contrary, all that the healings at Lourdes showed was that medicine had underestimated the power of the mind to heal the body. Alongside the power of suggestion, Bernheim now said, medicine needed to recognize a *second*, more potent power of the mind that was perhaps stimulated by religious belief but had itself no inherent religious

---

9. Georges Bertrin, "Notre-Dame de Lourdes," *The Catholic Encyclopedia*, vol. 9 (New York: Robert Appleton, 1910), accessed July 14, 2015, http://www.newadvent.org/cathen/09389b.htm.

implications. He called it "faith." "Faith moves mountains, faith performs miracles, because faith is blind, because it does not reason, because it suppresses control and impresses itself directly upon the imagination, without moderating second thoughts."[10]

Almost a century later, the journalist Norman Cousins described a remarkable cure — one that his doctors would have deemed impossible — in the pages of the *New England Journal of Medicine*.[11] He did not ascribe the cure to the grace of God, however. Prayer had played no role in it. What had cured him, he believed, was the power of his own mind; and, most important of all perhaps, a strong conviction in the possibility of his own cure. Was it really possible that a positive attitude itself could produce dramatic healings in this way? Was there any prior evidence? In asking these questions, Cousins invoked the object lesson of Lourdes. But then he suggested that the apparently miraculous healings seen there were neither more nor less miraculous than his own, and that perhaps there was a common explanation for them all: not the power of faith but the power of the placebo effect.

> It is quite possible that . . . everything I did . . . was a demonstration of the placebo effect. If so, it would be . . . important to probe into the nature of this psychosomatic phenomenon. At this point, of course, we are opening a very wide door, perhaps even a Pandora's box. The vaunted "miracle cures" that abound in the literature of all the great religions, or the speculations of Charcot and Freud about conversion hysteria, or the Lourdes phenomena — all say something about the ability of the patient, properly motivated or stimulated, to participate actively in extraordinary reversals of disease and disabilities.[12]

Was the placebo effect the key to making sense of all apparently miraculous healings, past and present? In the mid-1970s, two events unfolding within a few years of each other seemed to give some credence to this view. The first was an outgrowth of the discovery in the early 1970s of endorphins: substances in the brain that are chemically similar to opioids and that therefore appeared to be the brain's own natural painkillers. In 1978, a report was published that suggested that placebo treatments for pain were mediated, at least in part, by those biochemical substances. When an opioid-blocker called naloxone was used

---

10. Cited in Harris, *Lourdes*, 350.

11. Norman Cousins, "Anatomy of an Illness (as Perceived by the Patient)," *New England Journal of Medicine* 295 (1976): 1458–63.

12. Cousins, "Anatomy of an Illness (as Perceived by the Patient)."

to block the body's opioid receptors (without telling patients this was being done), placebo responders stopped reporting relief of pain.[13] Was there a real biochemistry to placebo responses and, by extension, to the power of positive thinking after all, just as Cousins had predicted?

The second event from the 1970s that began to transform the placebo from a suspect instrument of suggestion to a catalyst for the miracle cures of positive thinking was the rise of the new field of psychoneuroimmunology. In 1975, the psychologist Robert Ader at the University of Rochester put a powerful immune-suppressing drug, cyclophosphamide, in saccharine water and fed it to rats. (His goal was to create a state of nausea in the rats and condition them to associate it with the sweet taste of the water; he had not originally realized that the drug also suppressed the immune system.) When his rats grew ill and began to die, he stopped offering them the tainted water and fed them just plain saccharine water. Nevertheless, they continued to grow ill and die.

Why was this happening? In the end, he and his colleagues concluded that the rats had somehow been conditioned to make a link between the taste of the saccharine water and the biochemical action of cyclophosphamide. Their immune systems thus continued to act as if they were still being suppressed by the drug, something that then-current understandings of the immune system denied was possible.[14] The results had not been expected, but, faced with them, Ader began to ask: Had he not in the end, with his saccharine solution, done nothing more than create a placebo version of cyclophosphamide and, in so doing, shown that placebos were truly potent, even to the point of being able to depress the immune system of a laboratory animal to fatal levels? And if they could depress the immune system, why should they not be able also to enhance it, perhaps to the point of effecting a cure that otherwise would not have seemed possible? In such a context, to talk about the biochemistry and physiology of a miracle seemed like less of an oxymoron than it might otherwise would have and, for some, like a very exciting prospect. In the exuberant words of one student of the phenomenon: "The placebo effect is the good news of our time. It says, 'You have been cured by nothing but yourself.'"[15]

13. J. D. Levine, N. C. Gordon, and H. L. Fields, "The Mechanism of Placebo Analgesia," *Lancet* 23, no. 8091 (1978): 654–57.

14. R. Ader and N. Cohen, "Behaviorally Conditioned Immunosuppression," *Psychosomatic Medicine* 37 (1975): 333–40.

15. Lorette Kuby, *Faith and the Placebo Effect: An Argument for Self-Healing* (San Rafael, CA: Origin, 2001).

Prayer versus Placebo: What Is at Stake?

For Christians in particular, committed to good news of a different sort, this kind of talk was sure to rankle. There was, however — or so it seemed — a way to challenge it. All one needed to do was demonstrate definitively that some healings were due to neither standard medical interventions nor the placebo effect, but due to something else again, something that might be supposed to be God. Moreover, it was proposed one could demonstrate such a mechanism by adopting a methodology that would allow one to distinguish between mental powers and spiritual powers, between effects that are merely due to the mind's ability to influence the body and effects that apparently cannot be due to either mind or body (and therefore must be due to something else). The methodology in question is one that was originally designed to control (among other things) for the unwanted influence of psychological factors when attempting to determine the independent efficacy of new drugs: the randomized, placebo-controlled clinical trial (RCT).

How would this methodology work when now applied to testing the efficacy of spiritual techniques of healing? To see, let us consider a few of the most influential of these studies. The first of these was published in 1988 by a cardiologist named Randolph Byrd. For this study, 393 patients who had been admitted to the coronary-care unit of the San Francisco General Hospital were studied. Patients were randomly assigned into two groups. One of these would be prayed for, and the other would not (though there was no attempt to stop family members and others from praying for the people in the control group, leading to all sorts of odd discussion about the effects of "background" prayer and comparative "prayer dosage"). The so-called intercessors or prayers responsible for providing prayers to the "active treatment" group were all self-identified born-again Christians who claimed to pray daily and to go to church. Their task was quite specific: to pray daily for the speedy recovery of the patients and for no complications. The results showed no difference in the speed of recovery between the two groups, but Byrd found that, on six out of twenty-six kinds of possible complications, the prayed-for patients did better on a statistically significant level than the controls, and the controls did not do better than the prayed-for groups on any of the twenty-six measures.[16] In 1999, a Kansas-based researcher, William Harris, claimed to have replicated Byrd's findings with a larger population sample, though his study did not reproduce

---

16. R. J. Byrd, "Positive Therapeutic Effects of Intercessory Prayer in a Coronary Care Unit Population," *Southern Medical Journal* 81 (1988): 826–29.

any of the specific measures of improvement found by Byrd but rather found improvement on other measures.[17]

The studies carried out by Byrd and Harris both focused exclusively on the health benefits of Christian prayer. In 1998, however, psychical researchers Fred Sicher and Elizabeth Targ published the results of a six-month double-blind study of spiritual healing on forty AIDS patients in the San Francisco Bay area that took a much more ecumenical approach. The interveners consisted of forty practicing healers who self-identified variously as Christians, Jews, Buddhists, Native American shamans, and graduates of bioenergetic schools. Each of them was given a photograph of an AIDS victim, including the person's first name and his or her blood counts. In this study, rather than asking God to heal these patients, the healers were directed to send positive healing energy, to direct an "intention" for health and well-being to the subject. The authors claim that the twenty AIDS patients who received the healing energy (without knowing they had been selected for such treatment) had "fewer and less severe new illnesses, fewer doctor visits, fewer hospitalizations, and improved mood," compared with the twenty patients in the control group who did not receive the energy.[18]

The Return of the Psychological

The RCT approach to studying spiritual healing defined *spiritual* as a term effectively synonymous with *inexplicable*. The studies I have reviewed were not about the extent to which a person's medical condition might be influenced by the knowledge that he or she was being prayed for and the possible placebo effects or stress-reducing effects that might result. On the contrary, it was widely agreed that if there was even a chance that blinding was imperfect and that therefore subjects may have known they were being prayed for, then the study should be deemed null, void, and a failure.[19]

In this sense, the prayer studies stood apart from all the other efforts to inves-

17. W. S. Harris, M. Gowda, J. W. Kolb, C. P. Strychacz, J. L. Vacek, P. G. Jones, A. Forker, J. H. O'Keefe, B. D. McCallister, "A Randomized, Controlled Trial of the Effects of Remote, Intercessory Prayer on Outcomes in Patients Admitted to the Coronary Care Unit," *Archives of Internal Medicine* 159 (1999): 2273–78.

18. Fred Sicher, Elizabeth Targ, Dan Moore, Helene S. Smith, "A Randomized, Double-Blind Study of the Effects of Distant Healing in a Population with Advanced AIDS," *Western Journal of Medicine* 169, no. 6 (1998): 356–63.

19. I. Tessman and J. Tessman, "Efficacy of Prayer: A Critical Examination of Claims," *Skeptical Inquirer* 24, no. 2 (2000): 31–33.

tigate the effects of religion on health, because they were less about healing and more about metaphysics. The question that interested them, above all, was not just *what helped* but also *who*, in the culture wars between the religious and the secular sectors of our society, *had the truth*. This is why the prayer studies were, for a time, widely discussed, not just within religion and health circles but also in forums concerned with alleged scientific evidence for the existence of God and the supernatural. This is why also the studies were often reviewed alongside discussions of the strong anthropic principle from physics (the idea that our universe is the product of intelligent life), discussions of alleged fundamental weaknesses in Darwinian evolutionary theory, and discussions of the theological implications of so-called near-death and out-of-body experiences.[20] Their concern from the beginning was not with what patients believed or experienced but with whether objective data could be gathered that challenged the reigning naturalistic worldview.

Then, something happened that changed the game. In 2005, the *American Heart Journal* published a paper reporting the results of a research team headed by Herbert Benson that had originally been widely touted as the definitive and methodologically most rigorous study of the effects of prayer on health to date. It involved close to two thousand patients in six hospital sites, and the design was as follows. A total of 604 cardiac patients undergoing surgery were told that it was possible that they would be prayed for (and possible that they would not be) and were then prayed for. And 597 patients were told that it was possible that they would be prayed for (and possible that they would not be) and were then not prayed for. A final group was told that people definitely would be praying for them, and this was done. Classical clinical end points defined by the Society of Thoracic Surgeons were used as outcome measures, and a rigorous statistical analysis plan was designed.

The implicit assumption of the design was that if blinded prayer was effective (prayer in which there was no possibility of a placebo effect operating), then unblinded prayer (prayer involving both God *and* the placebo effect) would be even more effective. It was not what happened. There was no difference in recovery between the first two groups; in this sense, the experiment had failed to confirm the independent effectiveness of prayer. There was, however, an effect seen in the people in the group who knew for certain that they were going to be prayed for: they did worse than the other two groups. In the words of the researchers: "*certainty of receiving* intercessory prayer was associated with a higher incidence of complications."[21]

---

20. See, for example, Patrick Glynn, *God: The Evidence* (Rocklin, CA: Prima, 1997).
21. H. Benson, J. A. Dusek, J. B. Sherwood, P. Lam, C. F. Bethea, W. Carpenter, S. Lev-

While the researchers in their 2006 report suggested, almost in passing, that the findings might have been due to chance, most analysts were not satisfied. In the wry words of an editorial that appeared in the same issue of the *American Heart Journal*:

> It is rather unusual to attribute a statistically significant result in the primary end point of a prospective, multicenter randomized trial to "chance." In fact, such attribution is antithetical to the very definition of what error and statistical certainty imply: that the worse outcomes are almost certainly related to the therapy and not the play of chance. If the results had shown benefit rather than harm, would we have read the investigators' conclusion that this effect "may have been a chance finding," with absolutely no other comments, insight, or even speculation?[22]

The investigators were reluctant to discuss the possible meaning of their unexpected findings, in part, it seemed, because one conclusion that could readily be drawn from those findings is that — even leaving open the question of independent efficacy — prayer was not unambiguously a benign intervention. What might make it less than benign, however, was the meaning that the patient imputed to the information that he or she was to be prayed for. As the author of the same editorial quoted above noted: "Approaching a patient to participate in a prayer study before a procedure could inadvertently alarm a patient, 'You mean I'm so sick that I might need prayer?'"[23]

Benson's data, in short, raised the possibility that patients could experience a *negative* placebo response to a prayer intervention. However, because his study — like all the randomized controlled trials of prayer — had been concerned not with the subjective *experience* of prayer but with the objective *outcome* of prayer, no one had thought about the possibility of this happening, and so everyone had ended up feeling caught out. The psychological had trumped other agendas, and as a result, pretty much all the steam went out of the effort to study

---

itsky, P. C. Hill, D. W. Clem Jr., M. K. Jain, D. Drumel, S. L. Kopecky, P. S. Mueller, D. Marek, S. Rollins, and P. L. Hibberd, "Study of the Therapeutic Effects of Intercessory Prayer (STEP) in Cardiac Bypass Patients: A Multicenter Randomized Trial of Uncertainty and Certainty of Receiving Intercessory Prayer," *American Heart Journal* 151, no. 4 (2006): 934–42.

22. M. W. Krucoff, S. W. Crater, and K. L. Lee, "From Efficacy to Safety Concerns: A STEP Forward or a Step Back for Clinical Research and Intercessory Prayer? The Study of Therapeutic Effects of Intercessory Prayer (STEP)," *American Heart Journal* 151, no. 4 (2006): 762–64.

23. Krucoff, Crater, and Lee, "From Efficacy to Safety Concerns," 763.

intercessory prayer — conceived, as it had been, as a metaphysical project. The last year to see the publication of any new empirical, peer-reviewed studies in this area was 2006. A 2009 meta-review of the existing literature (a Cochrane review) concluded: "we are not convinced that further trials of this intervention should be undertaken and would prefer to see any resources available for such a trial used to investigate other questions in health care."[24] Had the studies, from the outset, been framed differently, it is unlikely that this would have been the conclusion.

Conclusion: What Should We Think?

At the outset of this chapter, I suggested that, before we could be prescriptive in our thinking about spiritual healing, we needed first to be diagnostic; we needed first to see how — either explicitly or implicitly — spiritual healing was already being both defined and assessed in contemporary medical research and elsewhere. Prayer studies have served as my case study for coming to some conclusions about the general tenor of current thinking, and it will be interesting to see whether other kinds of studies of spiritual healing — perhaps some being carried out in cultural contexts other than the Anglo-American — destabilize any of these conclusions. What I see happening in the prayer studies is a vision of spiritual healing grounded in a kind of eliminative logic: if results cannot be explained in terms of the placebo effect, in terms of stress reduction, in terms of social support, or in terms of any other accepted psychological or psychobiological category, then we can conclude that we are in the realm of unknowable spirit, in the realm of God's ineffable power. *God's power begins (or at least can be witnessed) only where the power of the mind leaves off* and only in the abstract space of statistical trends rather than in any specific individual case.

In consequence — and this does seem like an important consequence — the subjective experience of those who are on the receiving end of prayer usually is seen not as a source of potential insight but a source of potential distraction to experts on the hunt for more objective clues of divinity. Or it is so perceived until something happens — as happened to Benson's group — that puts the issue of experience front and center again.

What would our studies look like, however, if we were to resist current tendencies to conceive of *placebo* and *prayer*, mind and spirit, as antagonistic terms

---

24. Leanne Roberts, "Intercessory Prayer for the Alleviation of Ill Health," *Cochrane Database of Systematic Reviews* 6 (2014), accessed September 7, 2015, EBSCOhost.

and indeed were to resist the larger appropriation of prayer into the science-versus-religion culture wars of our time? What if we were to imagine a new generation of prayer studies in which experience was just as important as outcome, meaning just as important as mechanism? An undertaking such as this may influence our prescriptive desire to develop new best-practice norms that serve not just metaphysical debates but also human beings in all their complexity, as they actually experience the world.[25]

25. For more on these issues, see Anne Harrington, "The Placebo Effect: What's Interesting for Scholars of Religion?," *Zygon* 46 (2011): 265–80.

Part Three

Philosophical Insights

7

Philosophy of Mind and Emergentism in Thought about Healing

Philip Clayton

U
p to now in this volume, we have been charting biblical, historical, neuroscientific, and psychological approaches to the phenomenon of spiritual healing. We have also reflected critically on the recent attempts to capture spiritual healing through the lens of medical investigation of recuperation after major operations. But by now, it may be becoming apparent that our topic of spiritual healing has deeper and more complex philosophical and moral dimensions than was obvious at the outset of this investigation, and that these issues have to be confronted if the full range of issues encoded in the topic of spiritual healing is to be dealt with satisfactorily. To these problems, therefore, we now turn.

Thus, though it may seem surprising to some that people interested in the topic of spiritual healing would wish to pay careful attention to complex and sophisticated contemporary work in the philosophy of mind, our investigation has now led us inexorably to this point of reflection. Indeed, the present volume works with the premise that theologians and others interested in this topic of healing *must* enter into close dialogue with the best of contemporary science and philosophy — and indeed, that much may be gained from such a dialogue. By eschewing the so-called warfare model of the religion-science relationship, the authors in this volume embark on a risky voyage of integration: a voyage that, if successful, will leave neither side unchanged. We set out on uncharted seas with the conviction that an understanding of the religious or spiritual life that is consonant with the results of the sciences is superior to one that is isolated from or stands in conflict with them. More simply, we set out because we have no choice: the credibility of spiritual healing in an age of science depends upon an account of religion that is not at loggerheads with current scientific results.

Each chapter in this volume focuses the debate on one particular dimension of the science-religion interface. In this chapter, the emphasis lies on scientific approaches to the study of mind and, in particular, on the conclusions that contemporary philosophers have drawn from those results. Although it will quickly become clear that leading philosophers have been forced to some rather skeptical conclusions concerning the possibility of spiritual healing, I shall argue that theirs is not the last word. The scientific evidence is compatible with a theologically powerful affirmation of the spiritual dimension of healing. The goal in these few pages is to sketch a path toward that affirmation — not by negating the results and methods of the sciences but by incorporating their justified conclusions and supplementing them where there are grounds for doing so.

Spiritual Healing from the Perspective of the Philosophy of Mind

In its contemporary form, the philosophy of mind represents, roughly, the intersection set between three major fields: neurophysiology and the neurosciences, cognitive psychology, and the metaphysics of mind.[1] To a somewhat lesser extent, one also finds important contributions from primatology, evolutionary theory, other areas of psychology (including introspective psychology), cultural studies, and the philosophy of science. The discipline's key question is this: How should mind be understood in light of the full range of data currently available to researchers and those who reflect on this research? If forced to absolute brevity, I would list nine major philosophical positions in the field today that respond to this question. Ordered along a rough spectrum from materialism to idealism, they are the following: eliminative or reductive physicalism; nonreductive physicalism; epiphenomenalism; dual-aspect monism; weak and strong emergentism; weak and strong dualism; panpsychism and other forms of idealism.[2]

---

1. One knows, of course, that in philosophy nothing is uncontroversial. Technically one would have to add qualifiers to virtually all the claims that follow, since somewhere there is a philosopher who would dispute almost every point. Nonetheless, for reasons of style and brevity, I have omitted most of the qualifiers. The reader is forewarned.

2. For recent introductions to the field see, *inter alia*, Ernest Sosa and Enrique Villa-nueva, eds., *The Philosophy of Mind* (Oxford: Blackwell, 2003); Stephen P. Stich and Ted A. Warfield, eds., *The Blackwell Guide to Philosophy of Mind* (Malden, MA: Blackwell, 2003); David J. Chalmers, *Philosophy of Mind: Classical and Contemporary Readings* (New York: Oxford University Press, 2002); David Cockburn, *An Introduction to the Philosophy of Mind*

Although the different positions are hotly debated, one undeniably finds a distinct preference within the neurosciences and mainline philosophy of mind for the various positions that fall under the headings of physicalism, (materialist) monism, and weak emergence. Philosophers of mind admit that other positions are represented in the field, but such views tend to be seen as outliers from the standpoint of the discipline as a whole. I shall return in due course to the reasons given in defense of this prejudice, since I judge it to be unjustified. Although advocates of the other positions do publish and read papers in reputable fora within the discipline, the dominant voices claim that such persons have other, nonphilosophical motivations for taking the positions they do. Perhaps — this is often the biggest reservation against them — they hold theological presuppositions that cloud their judgment; or perhaps (it is believed) they do not fully recognize the significance of recent results in the neurosciences and, more generally, of the methodology that underlies the natural sciences and that allows the sciences to play the foundational role that they play in the human quest for knowledge. (In the end, many would say, these are probably just two different faces of the same mistake.)

Perhaps, in the context of a collection on spiritual healing, the position of mainline philosophy of mind will be dismissed as mere metaphysical prejudice — or mere antimetaphysical prejudice, as some may wish to dub it. Certain excesses notwithstanding, I wish to insist, however, that this dominant position is the result of argument rather than mere dogma — and, indeed, of an extended argument that is in many respects compelling. According to the argument, scientists and philosophers are committed to advancing only theories for which one can provide strong evidence. By this I mean discursive evidence — evidence that (potentially) any human being could assess. Science represents a particularly good example for this (Peircean) theory of knowledge, since its knowledge claims can be and regularly are assessed by researchers regardless of their cultural presuppositions or religious beliefs.

What does this commitment mean for the study of mind? Mind as a metaphysical entity, mind as soul created directly by God, even mind as *res cogitans* (thinking stuff) in the sense of Descartes — all of these views are inaccessible to discursive, scientifically informed study of the sort I have just described. (One possible exception is mind understood as an emergent reality. Here the line

(New York: Palgrave, 2001); Tim Crane, *Elements of Mind: An Introduction to the Philosophy of Mind* (Oxford: Oxford University Press, 2001); Jaegwon Kim, *Philosophy of Mind* (Boulder, CO: Westview, 1998); Anthony O'Hear, ed., *Current Issues in Philosophy of Mind* (New York: Cambridge University Press, 1998); and, most pointedly, Daniel C. Dennett, *Consciousness Explained* (London: Penguin, 1993).

between science and metaphysics could in principle be crossed. I return to this approach below.)[3] At the very least, whatever mind is, it must correlate with states of the brain and central nervous system if it is to be accessible to intersubjective study in a scientific manner. Thus the study of the neural correlates of consciousness (NCC) represents an indispensable component of any scientific approach to the question of mind.

At this point, there is a certain parting of the ways among those who work on this question. Some think that the study of NCC provides some knowledge of a different type of natural reality that they call the mental. Some, with greater agnosticism, argue that NCC point toward a causal force that common sense calls consciousness but that otherwise eludes philosophical analysis. Thus Colin McGinn speaks of the "mystery" of consciousness.[4] Jerry Fodor put the point more provocatively in a *Times Literary Supplement* article: "Nobody has the slightest idea how anything material could be conscious. Nobody even knows what it would be like to have the slightest idea about how anything material could be conscious. So much for the philosophy of consciousness."[5] By far the majority position in the field, however, is that the NCC do not justify one in arguing for a "different kind of reality" at all. Everything that we know and can know is physical, by which they mean that it is a part of or derived from the one natural world that we inhabit. It is just that, not surprisingly, the phenomena associated with this immensely complex organ that we call the brain — with its 10^{11} neurons and some 10^{14} neural connections — still elude full scientific understanding. Eventually, it is generally believed, evolutionary biology, neuroscience, and cognitive psychology will provide us with a much greater knowledge of these phenomena, and at that time we will have a fuller understanding of what we now call mind. For now, the important thing is to avoid mystifying mental phenomena unnecessarily — for example, by introducing occult forces. Such moves can only handicap the ongoing pursuit of a full and accurate understanding of the phenomena we call mental.

---

3. Certain arguments based on the role of holism in the natural sciences also offer important mediating possibilities. See, for example, Michael Esfeld, *Holism in Philosophy of Mind and Philosophy of Physics* (Dordrecht: Kluwer Academic, 2001).

4. See Colin McGinn, *The Mysterious Flame: Conscious Minds in a Material World* (New York: Basic, 1999).

5. Jerry Fodor, "The Big Idea: Can There Be a Science of Mind?," *Times Literary Supplement*, July 3, 1992, 5–7.

Doubts about the Move to Metaphysics or Theology

One can now see why I warned at the outset that this chapter would be rather more skeptical of the notion of spiritual healing (SH) than some of its neighbors. If theories of a finite soul — or a conscious mental substance that brings about changes in the physical world — already lie beyond what most philosophers of mind think can be attributed to the natural order, then how much more emphatically will they be skeptical of theories that ascribe physical changes to the agency of an infinite divine being or to angels and other spirits?[6]

Presumably, many readers will resist the argument that, in light of the data, one is most justified in concluding that what goes on in instances of alleged SH is best explained, ultimately, in purely physical terms. Let me then grant that it is at least *metaphysically possible* that some other form of causality is at work in alleged cases of SH — a form of causality, perhaps, that is not comprehensible even in principle in terms of the network of physical causation. Philosophers of mind will nevertheless argue that the *best available* explanations are of the sort I am about to summarize. As they urge, we should be concerned primarily with *inferences to the best explanation*, not with what might or might not be metaphysically possible.[7] I leave it to other authors to offer their speculations on the metaphysical realms that this chapter leaves open and undiscussed, insisting only that the epistemic status of their suggestions be kept clearly in mind.

The best available explanations, according to most philosophers of mind, are those drawn from the natural sciences and the quantitative social sciences. This commitment inclines the discipline toward particular strands of the spiritual-healing literature and away from others. In a significant *American Psychologist* article, William Miller and Carl Thoresen point out correctly that one must look for "possible biological pathways" in interpreting the data on medicine and spirituality.[8] Philosophers of mind would be quick to add that what one

6. One of the major problems is that of *overdetermination*: the outcome is determined by the chain of physical causes *and* by some nonphysical agent or agents. In attempting to avoid the overdetermination objection, proponents typically fall into epiphenomenalism, on the one side, and a denial of the causal closure of the physical world, on the other. Both of these two latter positions raise some difficulties. If forced to choose, I would give up on causal closure.

7. See Peter Lipton, *Inference to the Best Explanation* (London: Routledge, 2004), and the application to science-religion issues in Clayton, "Inference to the Best Explanation," *Zygon* 32 (1997): 377-91.

8. See William R. Miller and Carl E. Thoresen, "Spirituality, Religion, and Health: An Emerging Research Field," *American Psychologist* 58, no. 1 (2003): 24-35.

encounters in medicine-and-spirituality studies are merely *correlations*; the data do not determine causal linkages. It may be that some of these correlations are not explicable in terms of contemporary biology and medicine. But, for the epistemic reasons that I described earlier, this fact does not justify simply jettisoning the medical sciences; it is an inducement to do more and better research.

Harvard historian of science Anne Harrington is a major proponent of more humanized approaches to medical healing.[9] Harrington stresses the need to provide a sense of *communion*, arguing that it is "less about a need for more therapy and more about a need for more communion, less about making well and more about making sense."[10] Patients are rightly concerned that their caregivers share in their search for meaning and their sense of what is meaningful. I agree with her assessment, which is supported by studies in medical anthropology showing a variety of positive functions of healing rituals across cultures. Much is still to be learned about the functions of healing rituals, and future medical science will be stronger as it begins to study and incorporate these functions. Where the problems crop up, it seems, is in the attempt to move from these functional correlations, which can be empirically supported, to metaphysical interpretations, which cannot.

I note in passing that the widespread use of approaches based on semiotics has made it *harder* to justify the move to metaphysics, not easier. It is true — as Storck, Csordas, and Strauss point out with regard to the Navajo — that healing always includes a "conceptual scheme."[11] But this fact, again, does not open the door to old-style metaphysical reflection, for it is the *function* of these conceptual schemes that concerns scientific researchers, not their correspondence to some ultimate reality, which lies beyond the grasp of scientific study. As long as one focuses on the centrality of functional explanations of healing, one will tend to give a more cautious reading of the phrase *the power of the mind*.[12] Clearly, there are some significant correlations between recovery rates and certain attitudinal

---

9. Anne Harrington, *The Cure Within: A History of Mind-Body Medicine* (New York: W. W. Norton, 2008).

10. Anne Harrington, "Uneasy Alliances: The Faith Factor in Medicine; the Health Factor in Religion," in *Science, Religion, and the Human Experience*, ed. James D. Proctor (Oxford: Oxford University Press, 2005), 287–307.

11. Michael Storck, Thomas J. Csordas, and Milton Strauss, "Depressive Illness and Navajo Healing," *Medical Anthropology Quarterly* 14 (2000): 591, quoting Jerome and Julia Frank. Cf. also Csordas, *The Sacred Self: A Cultural Phenomenology of Charismatic Healing* (Berkeley: University of California Press, 1994).

12. On the interplay of the two dimensions, see in this volume Howard L. Fields, chapter 4, pp. 88–92.

states as reported by subjects and as measured in their behavior by means of reliable instruments. But these correlations, again, do not justify an immediate jump to a particular metaphysics of mind as the best explanation for the data on the experience and control of pain.

Interim Conclusions

We have begun to trace how and why contemporary work in the philosophy of mind supports the explanatory efforts of some authors on the topic of spiritual healing but stands in opposition to others. Imaging studies in the neurosciences, correlational studies in cognitive psychology, functional studies in medical anthropology, and the anthropology of religion provide important data for understanding the so-called spiritual dimensions of healing. *But they do not directly justify a metaphysics or theology of healing.* Indeed, philosophers of mind are inclined to view such metaphysical or theological interpretations with a significant degree of skepticism.

The philosophy of mind community is perhaps most critical of claims on behalf of parapsychological phenomena. One does not need to argue that humans *could not possibly* possess the powers to heal "open cancers" in other persons through mental effort, as claimed, for example, by Lawrence LeShan in *The Medium, the Mystic, and the Physicist: Toward a General Theory of the Paranormal*.[13] Instead, many philosophers will argue first that there is a major difference between reliable empirical correlations (assuming for the moment that LeShan's correlations are reliable) and causal explanations. If the data support correlations between prayer or "clairvoyant reality" and physical healing, then we should accept that the two phenomena are probably correlated.[14] (Perhaps one might be pardoned for a certain skepticism about LeShan's claim that "almost anyone can learn" how to heal others in this fashion.) But, even when empirically confirmed, *correlations do not explain.* Causal explanations explain. Thus one should remain dissatisfied with LeShan's interpretation of parapsychological correlations, and especially with his ungrounded assumptions about the precise causality involved, until actual causal explanations are established. In the meantime, it is rational to continue testing the correlations, controlling for and modifying as many possible causal factors as possible, until more compelling data is available.

---

13. Lawrence LeShan, *The Medium, the Mystic, and the Physicist: Toward a General Theory of the Paranormal* (New York: Viking, 1974).

14. Cf. Lawrence LeShan, *Clairvoyant Reality: Towards a General Theory of the Paranormal* (Wellingborough, Northamptonshire: Turnstone, 1980).

Unfortunately, philosophers often treat the question of spiritual healing in more traditional religious contexts as if it were identical to parapsychology. The differences, which are significant, will concern us in the remaining pages. But *to whatever extent that theologians or religious believers make claims similar to parapsychologists*, one should treat their claims in similar fashion. The empirical data on correlations between religious beliefs, rites, and rituals, on the one hand, and medical or psychological healing, on the other, should be drawn from reliable studies and be accurately presented. Where causal explanations exist for at least some portions of this data, they should be given priority over LeShan-like speculations. And, above all, one must be cautious about overquick causal leaps from correlations to spiritual entities and causal powers.

The Task of Integration

How should theologians and religious persons who have an interest in spiritual healing (SH) respond to work in the neurosciences and philosophy of mind? We have seen that these fields are rather resistant to endorsing causal influences that exceed the grasp of the sciences, including appeals to anomalous, paranormal, or supernatural powers and causes. One might even wonder: Would it not be better for religious persons to dismiss such challenges to strong theological accounts of SH? Perhaps religious discussions of spiritual healing should focus exclusively on presenting supporting data from the social sciences and from personal experience and then supplement them with straightforwardly theological interpretations and affirmations. This would mean that one would work exclusively with data consistent with religious assumptions, on the one hand, and with the language of one's particular faith tradition, on the other. Without a doubt, such a strategy would tend to promote more vibrant and more traditional theories of SH. Certainly it would make things easier.

But I fear that the problems are deeper than can be solved by this particular strategy. It appears that the generally accepted methodological standards — as well as a number of the central conclusions, not only in the neurosciences and philosophy of mind but also in many of the disciplines represented in this book — stand in tension with SH, at least when the latter is understood as the effect of special causes. Nor is it possible to subdivide the disciplines in which conflict arises, retaining an imagined empirical core while eliminating as merely ideological those portions that are skeptical of supernatural causes. There is no nonarbitrary distinction between the portions of psychology, sociology, anthropology, the neurosciences, the natural sciences, and for that matter contemporary philosophy that might be conducive to supernatural causes and the portions that are resistant to them. In each case, background assumptions, methods, theories, and results are much more organically connected. One can hardly chop off half a discipline and go on working with the rest, for disciplines generally depend upon methodological assumptions that bind together all work in the field. The rigor and predictive power of mathematical physics, for example, depends upon standards and criteria that serve to define what counts as a physical theory. To pick and choose among a discipline's conclusions based on criteria drawn from outside the field runs the risk of undercutting the discipline as a whole.

If disciplines cannot be subdivided in this fashion, then should religious believers challenge the validity of the disciplines as a whole, at least in their current form? Thus they might argue that the social sciences today are so compromised by their naturalistic assumptions that they can come to only false conclusions regarding SH. This strategy does not suffer from the inconsistencies that afflict the subdivide-and-conquer approach, but it does come with a price. For example, the wholesale rejection of social-scientific research on SH would tend to undercut the intellectual credibility of SH claims. One observes something like this result in the history of Christian fundamentalism in the United States:[15] cut off (by choice) from the support that the sciences, philosophy, and religious studies might have offered them, adherents have struggled to make a case for their beliefs that is persuasive beyond the parameters of a given religious group. Advocates of SH face a similar danger: excluding the social-scientific studies of SH would cut them off from important resources that might otherwise shed light on the very phenomena in which they are interested. Discarding the tools of the social sciences leaves one unable to answer serious intellectual objections that will inevitably be raised about SH, which in the long run may well undercut even the insider's sense of the viability of SH. By contrast, doubts and objections might be overcome *if one could integrate one's view of SH with the best current work from within the various relevant sciences.* It therefore seems crucial that one find a way to utilize all the various disciplines that bear on the understanding and assessment of SH — even if doing so requires one to deal explicitly with the challenges that these disciplines raise.

It is important to note in passing that the attitudes of authors writing on SH do not necessarily coincide with the official stance of the disciplines in which

15. See Martin E. Marty, ed., *Fundamentalism and Evangelicalism* (Munich: K. G. Saur, 1993), also Paul Anthony Schwartz and James McBride, *Fed Up with Modernity: Neo-Fundamentalism and the Christian New Right* (Berkeley: University of California Press, 1981); David O. Beale, *In Pursuit of Purity: American Fundamentalism since 1850* (Greenville, SC: Unusual Publications, 1986).

they were trained — a fact that is as true of the authors in this volume as it is of scholars in general. Authors trained in disciplines that are generally highly skeptical of healing claims sometimes offer vehement arguments on behalf of SH; in Britain one thinks, for example, of the neuroscientist Peter Fenwick and the cognitive psychologist Fraser Watts.[16] By contrast, although one would expect theologians to be uniformly positive about miracle claims, the present volume includes work by several professional theologians who take a much more cautious approach to the question of spiritual healing.

Two Major Approaches to the Question of Healing

At this point, one may have become skeptical about the possibility of integrating spiritual healing with results from the social sciences, the neurosciences, and the philosophy of mind. In order to assess the prospects, I return to the discipline with which this chapter began. Philosophers of mind are committed to the attempt to understand mind in light of the full range of data bearing on the subject. Hence they are required to include scientific data as well as narratives told by religious believers and healers. For example, in the Pentecostal movement worldwide, and in the movement of charismatic revival in the West, one finds widely circulated stories about miraculous healings, some of which include stories about people being raised from the dead.[17]

The problem, for a neutral observer, is not that some of these claims lie outside the ordinary experience of men and women today but rather that the overall data set concerning mind is inconsistent. The neurosciences and cognitive psychology have achieved significant empirical results and produced powerful explanations; yet they tend to rest on the methodological assumption that supernatural healings do not occur. Faith-based world views, by contrast, which generally retain a place for direct divine interventions, have a rather more difficult time integrating their causal claims with the mind-set and results of contemporary science.

---

16. See the papers collected by Fraser Watts and Geoff Drumbeck, eds., *Head and Heart: Perspectives from Religion and Psychology* (West Conshohocken, PA: Templeton, 2013), as well as the preface and conclusion by Watts; see also Fraser Watts, ed., *Spiritual Healing: Scientific and Religious Perspectives* (Cambridge: Cambridge University Press, 2011), esp. Watts's final chapter, "Concluding Integration." For an example of Fenwick's work, see Peter Fenwick and Elizabeth Fenwick, *The Art of Dying* (London: Continuum, 2008).

17. See the classic and highly influential text by John L. Sherrill, *They Speak with Other Tongues* (New York: McGraw Hill, 1964).

The entire discussion seems to boil down to two major approaches. On the one hand, one can begin with the premise that miracles (direct divine interventions) occur and then affirm only those parts of science that are consistent with this premise, doubting the rest. On the other hand, one can start with the sciences and then seek to find a nonarbitrary opening for SH — that is, a way of interpreting healing claims such that they remain at least consistent with the more fundamental results of the sciences (though not with the prejudices of all scientists).

I recommend the latter approach. It can be defined and characterized by four key requirements for an adequate theory of SH:

1. Requests for explanations of phenomena in the natural world are best met by causal explanations.

2. The need for causal explanations means that we should give preference to reconstructible causal histories. That is, the explanatory ideal is set by accounts in which the entire causal history can be traced and verified, at least in principle, by independent observers.

3. This criterion requires one to accept a certain presumption in favor of naturalism. Explanations are rationally assessable in this sense only when they involve causal histories that are found within the one natural world. Of course, *presumptive naturalism* is importantly different from *dogmatic naturalism*, for its naturalism is a methodological starting point that can be set aside if one later encounters compelling reasons to do so.

4. Finally, the view that I shall defend acknowledges that there are important interconnections among the various disciplines that study the natural world. Nonetheless, it emphasizes that not all explanatory interconnections need be reductive; they need not presuppose an ultimate reduction down to physics as the sole ultimately adequate framework for explaining all events in the natural world. Instead, the various disciplines are presumably connected in (roughly) the order in which their subject matters evolved over the course of cosmic history. As a result, one obtains the well-known hierarchy running from microphysics through chemistry and the increasingly complex levels of biology, and on to the study of human individuals and societies, culture, philosophy, and art. Levels that emerged later supplement earlier ones, though they remain in important senses dependent on them. Thus the earlier levels (say, the biological sciences) are not by themselves sufficient for explaining emergent phenomena (say, human social interactions). I shall use the term *emergentism* to refer to this position.

These four features function, I suggest, as *core working assumptions for an adequate study of human persons*, that is, a study that incorporates both scientific results and the *novum* that distinguishes our species from other life forms. To take one example, the goal of the neurosciences is to find out how far one can go in reconstructing the causal mechanisms that underlie those behavioral manifestations that we call consciousness or the first-person perspective. This is a plausible project, since there are overwhelmingly compelling reasons for accepting strong correlations between neural states and conscious states, and recent years have seen major progress in establishing the neural correlates of consciousness.

Still, the neuroscientific project does not require one to assume that consciousness is *nothing more than* a redescription of the neural states on which it depends. There are correlations between the air pressure in your tires and the miles per gallon that your car travels, but many other factors also affect the fuel efficiency of your car — including the personality attributes and mental state of the driver. Your genes influence your behavior, but so do cultural and historical factors that are trans- or epigenetic. Of course, one can decide to treat as real only those factors that can be counted, measured, or deduced from empirical laws and antecedent causes. But that is a decision, not an argument.

The Spiritual Dimensions of Healing

What notion of spiritual healing might be consistent with this methodological commitment? What disciplines and what topics might help one to formulate an understanding of SH that does justice to them? A number of possibilities come to mind, all of which are represented in the present volume: hermeneutics (John Swinton), cultural anthropology (Thomas Csordas), medical anthropology (Anne Harrington), and the study of patients' pain narratives (Howard Fields, among others). Consider just the final example: one can honor the narratives told by a Navajo participant in the Lightning Way ceremony, or those told by an English hospital patient who is involved in a charismatic healing service, without being committed to the literal truth of all the causal claims made about what occurred there. Indeed — though I do not myself share this degree of skepticism — one *could* endorse the narrative approach to SH in these two cases while believing that *all* the causal factors that influence illness and health in patients are in fact purely physical. The reason is one that professional social scientists are intimately aware of: spiritual beliefs can have positive functions without being true. Holding false beliefs — even about the causes of one's own healing — can have a positive influence on one's health, as the well-known studies of placebo effects clearly show.[18]

We return later to the question of the truth of the narrators' beliefs. For now, the crucial point is the possibility of separating the study of positive functions from the question of what is ultimately true in most, if not all, hermeneutical and social-scientific studies. Recognizing the importance of this separation-in-principle forces one to distinguish between two different approaches to the question of healing, which (following others in this book) I shall designate with the contrasting labels: *spiritual healing* and *the spiritual dimension of healing*. The term *spiritual healing* in what follows stands for the view that these healings involve their own type of causality, either supernatural or paranormal, as in the standard accounts of theology and parapsychology, respectively. The term *spiritual dimension of healing* (SDH), by contrast, need not entail that the healings involve supernatural or paranormal causal powers; it leaves open the possibility that they involve only natural causes, that is, causes that are amenable in principle to natural or social-scientific study. Advocates of SDH may, of course, insist that talk of a spiritual dimension is crucial for a full understanding of this type of healing. But they insist that the spiritual dimension may be incorporated in ways other than through the activity of paranormal or supernatural causes. Indeed, they often hold that explanations that eschew nonnatural causes may be crucial even (or perhaps especially) in cases where the individuals involved in the healing are themselves convinced that supernatural causes are involved.

Much turns on the difference between the two positions. SDH is certainly the less controversial of the two in most academic circles. Although it may encompass more, in its more minimalist versions it asserts only that persons are highly complex psychophysical systems who exist in complex interrelated social systems, systems that in turn depend on certain cultural and linguistic conventions that influence their members. Spiritual healing, by contrast, stands in greater *prima facie* tension with the natural sciences of our day — even if, in the end, these tensions can be overcome. From the perspective of the philosophy of mind with which this chapter opened, the existence of that tension must be acknowledged as a clear cost. It thus remains for us to inquire: Is the cost so great that it should determine the decision between the two approaches?

18. See, for example, Anne Harrington, ed., *The Placebo Effect: An Interdisciplinary Exploration* (Cambridge, MA: Harvard University Press, 1997), and Irving Kirsch, ed., *How Expectancies Shape Experience* (Washington, DC: American Psychological Association, 1999).

The Question of Top-Down Causation

The debate between SH and SDH is a debate between horizontal and vertical approaches to the question of healing and to the definition of those phenomena that we call spiritual.[19] As a first approximation, vertical approaches are those that retain language of God, divine influences, or supernatural powers; horizontal approaches either dispense with such language altogether or reinterpret it as expressing features of human existence, human society, or the human spirit. On this (loose) definition, Aquinas, Luther, and Barth come out as vertical thinkers, whereas Marx, Nietzsche, Feuerbach, and Freud are horizontal thinkers.

It turns out, however, that the distinction is not black-and-white, either-or. Consider, for example, the question whether spiritual healing involves a top-down dimension. Of course, some SDH explanations simply exclude the language of top-down altogether, parsing all analyses of healing in terms of the personal and interpersonal factors involved. But, I suggest, matters are more complicated than the simple dismissal of all vertical language would imply. Top-down causation, it turns out, comes in many shapes and sizes. The influence of a force field on the behavior of atoms is not the same as the influence of cell functioning on gene expression, which is not the same as the influence of the actions of individuals within a species on the subsequent development of that species' genome, which is not the same as the influence of population dynamics on the behavior of an individual animal, which is not the same as the influence of neocortical activity on hormone release or language use. None of these forms of top-down influence are identical to the apparent influence of thought on the brain, and mental causation in turn is not identical to the possible influence of God on the world.

Recognizing the immense variety of forms of top-down causation in the world — as emergence theorists have — cuts several ways.[20] It problematizes those discussions of healing that attempt a blanket exclusion of the vertical dimension in favor of purely horizontal accounts. But it also undercuts the widely used strategy of castigating one's opponents — those who do not accept one's own particular version of top-down causation — as only bottom-up thinkers or reductionists. If, as the evidence suggests, the variety of top-down influences is indeed greater than we formerly thought, then it is up to each scholar to give the best defense she can offer for the particular type of top-down causality that her

19. Ursula Goodenough, "Vertical and Horizontal Transcendence," *Zygon* 36 (2001): 21–31.
20. Harold Morowitz, *The Emergence of Everything: How the World Became Complex* (Oxford: Oxford University Press, 2002). For a brilliant analysis and defense of top-down causation, see George Ellis, *How Can Physics Underlie the Mind? Top-Down Causation in the Human Context* (Heidelberg: Springer, 2016).

account countenances.[21] Each participant in the discussion of spirituality and healing must defend, on the one side, her choice to *affirm* types of causes denied by her more cautious colleagues and, on the other, her decision to *deny* or *doubt* causes of healing that her less cautious colleagues affirm.

It would be interesting to locate authors on spiritual healing (say, those in the present volume) along a spectrum, based on their particular understanding of the vertical dimension in healing. I hypothesize that each author's readiness to affirm extraordinary types of causal influence will be in direct and inverse proportion to how costly he or she thinks it is to set aside, or at least supplement, the results of the natural sciences. The hypothesis would be easy to test with a simple questionnaire and some follow-up interviews. On the one end would lie those who endorsed the position, "I would not set aside the clear results of science at any cost"; these would presumably be the ones who are the most skeptical about claims for supernatural spiritual healing. At the other end would be those who respond, "There *is* no cost, or at least no serious cost, in setting aside the results of science"; perhaps they would add in explanation, "science is merely the expression of a series of assumptions and value commitments and hence represents a worldview of its own." For advocates of this science-as-worldview position, conflicts between science and (say) the religious belief that God heals persons need not be resolved in favor of science; there may be compelling reasons, they would presumably argue, for setting aside the methods and results of science. Others, closer to the middle, would nuance their responses: perhaps the core results of science cannot be rationally denied, but the interpretation of scientific theories and results (they might argue) leaves open the possibility of some degree of divine influence, which represents what we call the spiritual dimension in healing. My own answer to the questionnaire, at any rate, would lie in this direction.

Conclusion: Toward a Theology of Healing

Obviously, strong claims on behalf of spiritual healing are easier to defend when one denies science any epistemic privilege. If physics and theology are equal forms of knowledge, then scientific claims and miracle claims are on a par. But,

21. For more reasons to think that it is greater, see Clayton, *Mind and Emergence: From Quantum to Consciousness* (Oxford: Oxford University Press, 2004); Cynthia Macdonald and Graham Macdonald, eds., *Emergence in Mind* (Oxford: Oxford University Press, 2010); and Antonella Corradini and Timothy O'Connor, eds., *Emergence in Science and Philosophy* (New York: Routledge, 2010). For an opposing view of emergence, see Terrence W. Deacon, *Incomplete Nature: How Mind Emerged from Matter* (New York: W. W. Norton, 2012).

I suggest, there are weighty reasons to doubt the claim of epistemic parity. The precise mathematical predictions of the natural sciences, their high degree of intersubjective testability, their uncanny success at eliminating inadequate explanations and at converging on adequate ones suggest that they offer a uniquely rigorous form of knowledge. (To claim that science is the *only* form of knowledge humans possess is too silly to require refutation.) Consequently, where other claims to knowledge conflict outright with these results, we have *prima facie* a stronger reason to side with the science. Fortunately for theism, I think the conflicts are less frequent, and less essential, than is often claimed.

What about the belief that there is a supernatural dimension in some cases of human healing from physical or psychological illness? If this claim stands in essential conflict with science, then by the criteria we have developed, it should be viewed with some skepticism. But I believe that conclusion to be mistaken. The question of spiritual healing calls for a more nuanced — and hence a more interesting — response than such a blanket dismissal would allow. These final paragraphs attempt to sketch one such response.

The first step is to distinguish the epistemic parameters that we have discussed from the debate concerning viable metaphysical options. After all, accepting an epistemic presumption in favor of scientific explanations does not show that all metaphysical explanations are false but only that, in cases of direct conflict, the scientific account should be preferred. Knowledge questions have so far played a central role in our discussion of SH, and rightly so: one wants to know whether there is good reason to believe that spiritual healing actually occurs, or whether SH is merely a metaphor for purely natural processes of the sort that scientists study. What I wish to suggest is perhaps radical and unusual: that one should turn to the metaphysics or the constructive theology of healing not as an escape from the epistemic challenge of science but in response to and guided by it. Let the theologian ask not, "How can I develop a theology of healing to compete with the scientific limitations?" but rather, "Is there a robust theology that is consistent with the results we have obtained? Can one formulate a theology of healing that, working with the constraints of scientific knowledge, still offers a more-than-metaphorical account of what occurs in spiritual healing?"

The metaphysical starting point for such a theology of healing, I propose, is *panentheism* — the belief that the world is contained within God, although God is also more than the world. It is not that classical theology lacked a doctrine of the immanence of God: Christian theology has always stressed the closeness of God to God's creation. The trouble is rather that many of the philosophical resources that were developed for *thinking* about the immanence of God turned out in the end to work against the very thing they sought to protect. Conceptions of the God-world relation based on the notion of substances got in the way because relations between substances were understood to be *external* to those substances rather than internal to them. The perfection of the divine substance, therefore, came to mean that God could not be affected or changed by the world in any way and hence could not respond to creatures' suffering or prayers; the power of God came to be understood as coercive rather than persuasive, and so forth.

Panentheists in the nineteenth and twentieth centuries, therefore, turned to a different set of conceptual resources in attempting to reconceive the God-world relation. Major panentheistic proposals have arisen out of modern European idealism, process metaphysics, personalist understandings of reality, and conceptual resources drawn from non-Western religious traditions.[22] In the case of some process thinkers, panentheism may have emerged primarily in response to a philosophical framework (Whitehead's metaphysics) that the authors find superior to its competitors. For others of us, however, concern with the problem of divine action has provided the primary motivation for advocating panentheism. We have argued that panentheism represents the best conceptual framework currently available to theologians for conceiving divine action in the world in a manner that is fully compatible with the scientific account of nature.

Consider, for example, the panentheistic analogy.[23] The analogy suggests that, for those who seek to clarify God's relationship to the world, analogies with the relationship of our minds to our bodies can be helpful. (I leave it to the reader to add in the obvious respects in which these two relationships are different.) On what I take to be the most credible understanding of mental phenomena, mind is not identical to the body; our mental experience represents and responds to states of the body and its changes, but it also includes an element of awareness that goes beyond the state of any individual part of the body. Moreover, our mental states also have effects on the actions our bodies take. Thus, for example, my awareness that what I *really* want is to graduate from college, rather than (say) to get more sleep or to play professional football, causes me to carry out

22. For an excellent overview of the core tenets of panentheism, see Michael Brierley, "Varieties of Panentheism," in *In Whom We Live and Move and Have Our Being: Scientific and Theological Perspectives on God and World*, ed. Philip Clayton and Arthur Peacocke (Grand Rapids: Eerdmans, 2004), and other essays in the same volume. See also Loriliai Biernacki and Philip Clayton, eds., *Panentheism across the World's Traditions* (New York: Oxford University Press, 2013), and Philip Clayton, *Adventures in the Spirit: God, World, Divine Action* (Minneapolis: Fortress, 2008), esp. part 3 on panentheism.

23. See Philip Clayton, *God and Contemporary Science* (Grand Rapids: Eerdmans, 1997), ch. 8.

different actions in the world than I would were I not guided by this overarching mental state. Yet there is certainly nothing abnormal or nonnatural about one's mind responding to one's body and in turn influencing its actions: every word we speak and every conscious action we take bears witness to the unproblematic nature of this connection.

For panentheists, the relationship of God and world is (in a few crucial respects) analogous to the above. Panentheists do not conceive God dualistically, as separate from the world, such that it would take a divine incursion into the world in order for God to be associated with inner-worldly happenings. After all, this is precisely the picture that led to the so-called warfare model of science and religion through much of the modern period.[24] Rather, God's response to the existence of creatures — their hopes, aspirations, and sufferings — is as natural and immediate as the mind's response to the body. And God's ability to direct creaturely responses is as immediate and natural as the mind's involvement in specific bodily responses. In fact, one might say that panentheism has the problem opposite to that of classical philosophical theism (CPT): if CPT had first to establish how a divine influence on finite substances was possible, panentheism needs to specify how it is that we can attribute causal agency to finite things — is not *all* agency in the end God's agency?[25]

But what of the obvious disanalogies between finite minds and the divine mind? The epistemological perspective defended in this chapter suggests that one should not attribute to human minds powers and abilities that are in conflict with what we know to be physically, chemically, and biologically possible. Yet why should God be limited by such constraints? The theology of *kenōsis* or the self-limitation of God is helpful in addressing this question. Although even

24. The warfare model was advocated, for example, by Charles T. Gorham in *Religion as a Bar to Progress* (Girard, KS: Haldeman-Julius, 1944). For detailed histories of the interactions between science and religion, see David C. Lindberg and Ronald L. Numbers, eds., *God and Nature: Historical Essays on the Encounter between Christianity and Science* (Berkeley: University of California Press, 1986); David C. Lindberg and Ronald L. Numbers, eds., *When Science and Christianity Meet* (Chicago: University of Chicago Press, 2003); John Hedley Brooke, *Science and Religion: Some Historical Perspectives* (Cambridge: Cambridge University Press, 1991); John Hedley Brooke, *Of Scientists and Their Gods* (Oxford: Oxford University Press, 2001); John Hedley Brooke and Geoffrey Cantor, *Reconstructing Nature: The Engagement of Science and Religion* (New York: Oxford University Press, 2000).

25. Again, I separate classical philosophical theism from the scriptural statements about God's involvement with the world and from the core intentions of theologians of (say) the patristic period. The problem lies not in the *intentions* of the theologians but rather in the philosophical framework many used to try to conceive the biblical picture of the relationship between God and world.

from a panentheistic perspective it remains metaphysically possible for God to act at any instant in such a way that God sets aside well-known physical and biological limitations, God, in fact, seems to work within the structures of the natural world as God established it — presumably because this is the only way for natural creatures with their own free agency to evolve. Thus one should say that, although God has the capacity in principle to heal bodies and minds in ways that contradict all physical possibility, God appears to work within the constraints of the natural order (once it has been established) by guiding, directing, and luring the created universe in a manner consistent with its inbuilt laws and regularities.

So is there then nothing for God to do? Is the word *God* merely a pleasant metaphor for what are in the end purely physical, biological, and psychological causal processes? Our discussion of mental influence using the panentheistic analogy suggests a rather different conclusion. If one accepts the existence of a divine being, it is *plausible* to hold that God plays a role *not less active and intimate* than the influence of mental states on the body with which they are associated. Human concentration and will can bring about bodily actions that would otherwise not have occurred, and we have good evidence that psychological states can influence the healing process in ways not yet explicable at the physiological level alone (see essays elsewhere in this volume and the literature cited therein). Thus one can only imagine that the potential for divine causal influence within the world — even an influence that, because of divine self-limitation, remains completely consistent with the established causal order of nature — is at least as great.

One must ask, finally, what *type* of divine influence can most plausibly be postulated and where one might expect to see it at work. The conflict with science is the greatest for those who imagine that God directly alters outcomes in *purely physical causal systems*, since science's knowledge and predictive powers are greater for such systems than for any other domain in our experience. It is, therefore, more expensive epistemologically to assert that God directly and immediately alters the path of a falling boulder as it careens down the hill toward a house than to make almost any other statement one might possibly make about the divine. The frontal challenge to scientific methods and results is only somewhat less grave in the case of direct alterations of chemical and biological systems, however. To argue that God dissolves millions of bacteria in an infected body without the mediation of antibodies or medications directly undercuts the possibility of medical science as we know it today, as well as the free will of organisms themselves.

By contrast, an influence of God on the mind — that is, on the complex of mental properties and psychological states that emerges from the brain and central nervous system without being reducible to them — is a different matter altogether. We have good reason to think that the human mental life is not reducible to a set of laws, a position that the philosopher of mind Donald Davidson has defended under the heading of "anomalous monism."[26] Thus we have reason to think that no natural laws would be broken were God to comfort a person, strengthen her resolve, or hold out ideals for action. (Were the presence of the divine to compromise or overcome her very sense of personhood, her ability to act as an autonomous agent, one would face a very different type of problem.)

Consequently, it is here, at the level of human mental causation, that one can most plausibly locate one's account of divine influence in cases of spiritual healing. Whether God strengthens the will, resolve, and hope of the suffering person or whether God also helps set in motion latent healing powers of the mind not yet fully understood by science is unclear; perhaps both types of influence occur. If either form of divine influence takes place, one can say that spiritual healing occurs — and indeed, in a manner that involves both a real causal influence by God and a respect for the natural order as the sciences have revealed it to us.

Do we know that God never actually heals in any more direct, supernatural, and miraculous sense than this? No, one cannot exclude this possibility. Certainly it belongs to the nature of the divine to be capable in principle of exercising science-contradicting causal powers. And perhaps the eye of faith will discern such direct interventions either occasionally or on a regular basis. But if one excludes the heart's reasons "that reason knows not of," then, I suggest, one will never have *better* intersubjective reasons for asserting that such direct physical healing occurs than for concluding that a more indirect influence, an influence mediated through the mind, was involved. That the court of collective human knowledge cannot pass judgments that transcend this limitation on what can be rationally affirmed should come as no greater surprise to faith than it is to reason.

26. Donald Davidson, "Thinking Causes," in *Mental Causation*, ed. John Heil and Alfred Mele (Oxford: Clarendon, 1995), 3–17.

8

Healing and the Moral Problems of Efficacy

Stephen R. L. Clark

In the last chapter, Philip Clayton demonstrated how reflection on the topic of spiritual healing leads inexorably to the probing of certain philosophical questions, and especially those associated with the metaphysics of the mind/body relation, on the one hand, and the ontological relation of God to the world, on the other. But it is not just these big metaphysical questions that are summoned by our topic of spiritual healing. No less significant are the subtle problems of moral discernment and ethical judgment that are also implied by any careful examination of healing events, as disclosed in the field.

In order to get a handle on some of these issues of moral discernment and moral efficacy, I propose in this chapter to take a fresh look at the topic from the perspective of a remarkable late antique philosopher, whose insights may fruitfully be compared with those Christian authors who were profoundly influenced by him. Sometimes moral light comes from unexpected sources.

What's Spiritual about Spiritual Healing?

The principal focus of my own present work is the third-century philosopher Plotinus, who had an enormous influence on the theological and aesthetic tra-

This work was made possible by the award of a Major Research Fellowship by the Leverhulme Trust. My thanks to Sarah Coakley and other participants in the colloquium for their comments and advice, and to Gillian Clark.

ditions of Western and Eastern Christendom and on Islam. He is also widely considered to echo or even to have had some connection with the development of Indian philosophy. His work was edited, thirty years after his death, by his friend and disciple Porphyry of Tyre, who chose to dismember and distribute the text into six volumes, each with nine treatises (thus, the *Enneads*). By any plausible definition of spirituality, Plotinus was a spiritual teacher and one who had no high opinion of "spooky" methods of healing — both because he thought them ineffective and presumptuous and because he thought they misdirected our attention.[1] My contribution to the study of spiritual healing or the spiritual dimensions of healing is, therefore, skeptical but of a different order from the skepticism of modern materialistic philosophy of mind, as expounded by Philip Clayton. To explain how and why, I must first address some general conceptual issues.

What counts as spiritual healing or as the spiritual dimensions of healing? What is spiritual health or spirituality in general? This problem has exercised us throughout the pages of this book, but perhaps more can still be said by way of illumination. In ordinary discourse, spirituality seems to be a sort of "religion lite": those who think of themselves as spiritual or who wish for some spiritual element in their lives and in society usually profess concern for something more than merely material advantages, and they sometimes also believe in other sorts of explanation than the merely material (the term *material* itself having many meanings). They may describe spiritual experiences in which they felt themselves caught up in some exalted mood and hope that these experiences, or whatever reality lies behind them, may make them healthier, wealthier, or wiser. They may often seek to distance themselves from any established religious cult and deny the importance of any precise theological or metaphysical speculation or commitment. The merely religious are reckoned authoritarian and judgmental; the spiritual are tolerant of diversity (though not, as a rule, of any established religion) and prefer more private rites.[2] The merely religious may also, it is supposed, have fewer real or rational commitments, while spiritual people may be presumed to have some idea of what they are doing or feeling and why (despite their unwillingness to spell out their doctrines). Some spiritual teachings, of course, may be found even in the established religions and constitute a "spiritual core" (as some would say) of doctrine and practice. Ordinary

1. By *spooky* in this chapter, I intend the current colloquial albeit vague meaning — that is, uncanny, ghostly, weird, or mysterious.

2. For example, "spirituality . . . often seems to be a way of retaining the 'nice' bits of religion without having to face either the criticisms or demands of adherence to an organised religious tradition." Denise Cuse, "Engaged Religious Studies," *Discourse* 4, no. 2 (2005): 87.

believers may follow the outward rules, but true or spiritual believers see the real significance of those rules and follow them according to the spirit rather than the letter. This judgment could be questioned.

Health is at least as contentious a term. For some, health is merely the absence of overt disease or disability. For others (notoriously, the World Health Organization), "health is a state of complete physical, mental and social well-being and not merely the absence of disease or infirmity."[3] Even notions like disease or infirmity, let alone well-being, are contentious, especially but not only when their range is extended from the merely physical to cover mental, social, or, of course, spiritual processes. Modern moralists may unconsciously equate health with being comfortable, being able and inclined for ordinary pursuits, being sociable, or having at least an *average* life expectancy (so that a physically fit victim of Alzheimer's is, in a way, healthy and, in another way, not). Some even seem to think that children who are too lively or, alternatively, too quiet need medical intervention. This is at least a change from the days, not long ago, when young women judged to be "promiscuous" were imprisoned without appeal in mental hospitals.[4] Despite the heady ideals of the World Health Organization and social reformers, mainstream physicians are perhaps more likely to practice a more vulgar medicine: their goal must be to cure or alleviate particular diseases, disabilities, or deformities without regard to the ideal quality of their patients' future lives. Alternative practitioners — and even mainstream doctors in their more thoughtful moments — may profess a more personal and holistic care: what matters is the *patient*, not merely her medical condition. This concern, in turn, may seem to be more spiritual than the work of a harried general practitioner, required to identify and treat her patients' problems as calmly, professionally, *and quickly* as a car mechanic. To be healthy, some suppose, is to be *whole*. To be whole, in turn, is to be spiritually alert, alert to spiritual issues, and to be freed from merely conventional bonds or habits.

Most of these vague notions may now seem uncontroversial, however bad we are at putting them into practice. Who could deny that we should be concerned with the whole person or that spiritual health must heal the splits between soul and body, reason and emotion, the individual and the community? Who could deny that spiritual wisdom is needed to detect the signs and causes of spiritual sickness and that such sickness may lie behind the merely physical symptoms

3. So defined in the constitution of the World Health Organization, accessed December 20, 2018, https://www.who.int/about/mission/en/. See also Helen King, "What Is Health?," in *Health in Antiquity*, ed. Helen King (Abingdon: Routledge, 2005), 1–11.

4. See Maggie Potts and Rebecca Fido, *"A Fit Person to Be Removed": Personal Accounts of Life in a Mental Deficiency Institution* (Plymouth: Northcote House, 1991).

of overt disease or disability? Who could deny that convention is often a deadening influence? Those who feel these doctrines most strongly may sometimes suppose that they must espouse some nonmaterialistic metaphysics, but even metaphysical materialists may recognize the importance — if they can afford the time — of considering the social, psychological, and even philosophical contexts of overt disease and may acknowledge that some practitioners have a keener sense of these than others. Conversely, metaphysical idealists — supposing that the apparently material world is no more than the effect of nonmaterial causes — may still not be entirely persuaded that we are ever competent to judge these matters fairly and, therefore, prefer to consider merely physical conditions piecemeal without regard to their own or their patients' spiritual welfare.

Before we can achieve any clarity about spirituality, health, and spiritual health, at least three topics need to be distinguished: spiritual techniques of healing, the spiritual dimensions of healing, and spiritual health itself. Spiritual techniques of healing, especially in New Age circles, may include the use of crystals, feng shui, chakras, prayer, and the laying on of hands. Such things are spiritual, it may be supposed, because they do not rely on established biological or medical theories and practice and, perhaps, because they demand less violence than more ordinary means in their production or their testing. They also seem, as already acknowledged, "spooky": worrying intrusions on our everyday familiar world. Some of them may turn out to be less spooky than they seem. The occasional efficacy of the healing hand seems spooky — suggestive of entities or processes that mainstream medicine does not admit — as long as we suppose that it is the healer's hands that have some special virtue or that mystic energies are conveyed from healer to patient. Such energies would be mystic because they cannot be captured in a physical formula or equated with such and such an increase or decrease in temperature or electromagnetic emissions. But if the healing hand works simply because the *patient* is comforted by a professionally or personally friendly touch, and her biochemistry alters in response to this, the effect is wholly compatible with a properly physical understanding of the organism. Even more dramatic procedures, involving saliva or drum music or the apparent removal — by suction — of arrowheads or other sharp objects from a patient's body may have real effects, not because of any special energies but because we are all disposed to respond to these dramatic therapies. Even the recollection or imagination of past lives may have a therapeutic effect, regardless of whether those stories are veridical. These are sometimes referred to as placebo effects, but this is probably to misunderstand them: they do not work simply because the patient *believes* they will but because physical contact, music, drama, even outright fantasy have effects whatever we believe about them or even if we have no beliefs at all (babies are comforted by a touch or a lullaby but not because the baby *thinks* that these help her).

The stories we tell about ourselves and about the world have real effects, whatever truth they have. But of course, it may be difficult to take such stories seriously as therapy without beginning to suspect that they may also testify to a larger and stranger world than mainstream medicine admits. And other apparently successful techniques (for example, prayer) may seem positively to require some larger modification of mainstream scientific theory: perhaps minds are less localized than we suppose and can reach out somehow to a distant patient. It is sometimes suggested that even such events could be accommodated within mainstream science: after all, the phenomenon of quantum entanglement — whereby particles that were once associated somehow respond to each other's changes even at distances too great for travel between them to be possible — is both spooky and well-attested.[5] But it seems likely that this is no more than a metaphor: such quantum entanglements offer no plausible mechanism for the apparent efficacy of petitionary prayer. If such prayer does indeed work, then the traditional explanation, in terms of disembodied spirits or the priority of mind over matter, may seem to offer a more plausible story.

But consider one extremely spooky theory that would serve to explain such occasional effects and that has had support in recent years from unexpected sources. Maybe our present experience is indeed, as ancient philosophers have argued, a dream and a delirium. Maybe, in short, we are inhabiting a merely *virtual* reality, an entertainment or learning program controlled by advanced computers. The possibility of such virtual realities, well advanced from those entertainments that we already recognize, is real. The more likely we think it is that such programs will get more sophisticated and that computer power will continue to increase, the more probable we must suppose it is that *most* experiences, say, of early twenty-first-century life will be virtual ones.[6] What happens in the entertainment will be determined by the overall program of the computers and the expressed wishes of the players (some of whom, perhaps, have the appropriate passwords to override the programming, whether they know this or not). Of course, the more likely we think it is that this experience is only virtual, the less reason we have even to believe that the real world is much like the virtual; maybe we, our real selves, inhabit the end-time when all ordinary sources of energy have

5. For an accessible account of this phenomenon, see Brian Greene, *The Fabric of the Cosmos* (London: Penguin, 2004), 80–81.
6. The argument is developed by Nick Bostrom, *Anthropic Bias: Observation Selection Effects in Science and Philosophy* (London: Routledge, 2002).

been exhausted, and we rely instead on Hawking radiation from controlled black holes.[7] This world here, the world of our present experience, is one of indefinitely many fantasies or semihistorical psychodramas, and we may wake from it (as ancient philosophers also hoped) either at our seeming deaths or in a moment of revelation. Or perhaps we can go still further afield: the real world is nothing at all like the world we imagine, and all the entities and processes (including Hawking radiation) that scientists have postulated are merely further fantasies. Our seeming ancestors were closer to the truth in reckoning that the real world was a world of spirits and that we came here through a hole in heaven.

Suppose that this is so. Can we immediately say that this is a *spiritual* revelation? Certainly, it provides a neat metaphor for the ancient hope that we may wake from our delirium, and incidentally it shows the absurdity of denying the conceptual possibility of "surviving death."[8] But suppose that we, our real selves, have embarked on our entertainment out of terminal boredom. Suppose that we only expect to indulge emotions that have long been controlled or eliminated in the ultimate world. Or suppose, more honorably perhaps, that we are seeking the chance to practice *virtues* — of generosity, courage, or simple prudence — that cannot be exercised or felt in the real world.[9] On those last terms, it would be this world here that was the spiritually superior world, the one that allowed at least an imitation of virtue. The real world within which the program is running may be *ontologically* prior to this world but not *axiologically* (ranked by its worth). The dream would be better than waking, whether because it is more exciting or because it provides a better field for heroes.

Such a virtual world, of course, would still be a very unsatisfactory one. The virtues we exercise would be dependent on our self-deception, on our remaining convinced, falsely, that there are creatures in need or danger.[10] They would be no less

---

7. See George F. R. Ellis, ed., *The Far-Future Universe: Eschatology from a Cosmic Perspective* (Philadelphia: Templeton Foundation Press, 2002).

8. See my "Waking-Up: A Neglected Model for the Afterlife," *Inquiry* 26 (1983): 209–30.

9. In some real worlds, like that envisaged by Plotinus, virtue is all the better for *not* being put into practice: a truly courageous person, for example, would not actually want to display courage — since that depends on there being wrongs to resist or even wars to fight "as if a physician were to wish that nobody needed his skill" (*Enneads* 6.8 [39].5, 13–21). But that is not the sort of real world that is imagined here. Unless otherwise noted, all citations of the *Enneads* are from the translation of A. H. Armstrong (Plotinus, *Enneads*, 7 vols., Loeb Classical Library [Cambridge, MA: Harvard University Press, 1966–88]).

10. See *Enneads* 6.7.26, 20ff.: "Certainly the good which one chooses must be something which is not the feeling one has when one attains it; that is why the one who takes this for good remains empty, because he only has the feeling which one might get from the good. This is the reason why one would not find acceptable the feeling produced by something

counterfeit than the heady emotions that now attend our visits to a cinema; movie heroes are not real heroes, and the lift we get from participating in their seeming heroism is still less like real virtue. Plato was right in this at least, that such imitations are axiologically inferior. Augustine was in the same tradition, in judging his own past enjoyment of the theater harshly: "In my wretchedness I loved to be made sad and sought for things to be sad about: and in the misery of others — though fictitious and only on the stage — the more my tears were set to flowing, the more pleasure did I get from the drama and the more wonderfully did it hold me."[11]

If the story as I have told it is true, it is a truth not worth acknowledging, and all our judgments about values are suspect. Science itself would be a pointless game — pointless, that is, except in giving creatures who already *have* all the available answers a misleading sense of achievement in working out the answers (or the answers that the program lets them have) apparently for themselves. Clearly, we had better not believe this story — but not because it is demonstrably untrue. We had better not believe it because such a belief would sap our ethical and epistemic energies, for no obvious gain — though of course even that inference is untrustworthy. Good Platonists will insist instead that we should believe that reality is such as to make it possible, and probable, that we can and should attain to truth. For them, that is, what is ontologically prior is also axiologically prior — and this is a more stable theory than the hideous fable I have been sketching, one to which I shall return.

But the principal moral here is that a theory can be spooky without being spiritually healthy (or so at least it seems) and that not all imaginable occult truths would be worth knowing. Some such imaginable truths would remove all value, including the values of scientific inquiry and well-intended therapy. I suspect that all we should have to fall back on would be sensation, and our virtual realities would be revealed as little more than very hard-core porn. That would be deplorable if there were an axiologically higher reality, but not if we are merely actors in a virtual entertainment (comedy, horror, action, seeming tragedy, or farce).[12]

---

one has not got; for instance, one would not delight in a boy because he was present when he was not present; nor do I think that those who find the good in bodily satisfaction would feel pleasure as if they were eating when they were not eating or as if they were enjoying sex when they were not with the one they wanted to be with, or in general when they were not active."

11. Augustine, *Confessions of St. Augustine*, trans. F. J. Sheed (New York: Hackett, 1942), 37 [3.2]. Unless otherwise noted, all subsequent citations of the *Confessions* are from Sheed's translation.

12. For further commentary on this sort of possibility, see Glenn Yeffeth, ed., *Taking the Red Pill: Science, Philosophy and Religion in* The Matrix (Chichester: Summersdale, 2003).

The suggestion that I have slipped into this discussion is, implicitly, that the spiritual has something to do with ethics or with virtue or at least with value: the spooky world I described is not a spiritually superior world because it is, or easily might be, of much less worth than our own. *Spiritual* forces must be axiologically, not just ontologically, superior; that is why we speak of them as gods or as obedient agents of the one God. The computer programmers of my fantasy are not worthy objects of worship, even if we have some reason at least to be *wary* of them. Spiritual techniques of healing, unless they are closely linked to virtue and to value, are merely spooky — temporarily spooky, till we have discovered their place in a broadly physicalist theory, or permanently spooky if they intimate, for example, that we are living in a real dream. So the question is this: In exercising the healing arts, what dimensions are intended by reference to the spiritual?

One answer, already intimated, is that healers, doctors, medics, and nurses should take account of their patients as the human beings they presume they are. Where patients can express a view on the matter, their view should at least be listened to, and they should have some sense that they are being dealt with as human beings in a humane society. When they cannot, opinions may begin to differ. Some medical ethicists — and they seem at the moment to dominate public debate — propose that patients are owed this fundamental respect only as long as they are fully persons. If they cannot talk, reason, or respond unambiguously as fully conscious beings, they have, on the dominant account, no rights at all (except, perhaps and anomalously, the minimal right to be spared actual pain). More traditionally minded ethicists, claiming a greater spiritual sense, reject this view entirely. So John Paul II, in *Evangelium Vitae*, rebukes "the mentality which tends to equate personal dignity with the capacity for verbal and explicit, or at least perceptible, communication. It is clear that on the basis of these presuppositions there is no place in the world for anyone who, like the unborn or the dying, is a weak element in the social structure, or for anyone who appears completely at the mercy of others and radically dependent on them, and can only communicate through the silent language of a profound sharing of affection."[13] We should not treat patients, even patients whose lives seem to us or some of us to lack some essential element of a fully human life, as if they were merely pieces of broken machinery or animals to be put down to end their possible pains.[14] The spiritual dimension of healing, on this account, is simply

13. *Evangelium Vitae* (delivered March 25, 1995), accessed December 20, 2018, http://w2.vatican.va/content/john-paul-ii/en/encyclicals/documents/hf_jp-ii_enc_25031995_evangelium-vitae.html.

14. I should add that I do not myself suppose that even *animals* should be treated "like animals": the respect we owe to any of God's creatures should forbid us to treat them dis-

the humanistic dimension of healing with the added requirement that we *not* judge lives as not worth living merely because the patients cannot talk, reason, or perform some voluntary action. We should acknowledge, perhaps, their *spiritual* being even if their physical and mental capacities have been diminished or eliminated.

But in what does that spiritual being consist? If we accept that even the terminally infirm deserve our continued care and respect, does this require us to believe that they are actually, really, more than their mortal minds and bodies? If their bodies are irreparably damaged and their minds no longer capable of rational or personal response, what is there left of them? Must our treating them respectfully be no more than the residual (and perfectly proper) respect we give to human corpses (as every human society has done, since Neanderthals buried their dead with flowers)? Remembering their spiritual being would then be to incorporate them in a symbolic structure in which their damaged minds and bodies must be treated respectfully because they are images of the fully human, not because the persons that they were somehow still exist. We take care of them for our sake, not for theirs. Matteo Ricci, the sixteenth-century Jesuit missionary, offered a similarly expressive account of Chinese rituals that involved the presentation of food or drink to their ancestral spirits:

> They [the Chinese] do not believe that the dead will come to eat or even need these things. They say that there is no other way to express their love and gratitude to the dead. Some told me that these rituals are set up for the living people, not the dead — that is, to teach the children and the ignorant to respect their parents that are still alive. . . . In any case, they do not think that the people who are gone are gods or spirits, thus they do not pray for anything. It has nothing to do with idolatry. Hence it seems not to be superstition.[15]

Self-consciously modern but still sentimental therapists may find a similar excuse for caring for those they think are no longer persons. Alternatively, maybe the terminally infirm really do exist in some connection with their mortal frames and should be addressed directly even if they cannot — in this world — answer us. If that is so, then we must reconsider the dominant modern metaphysics

---

respectfully. But in this context, I am concerned solely with the spiritual dimensions of *human* health.

15. Matteo Ricci, *China in the Sixteenth Century: The Journal of Matteo Ricci, 1583–1610*, trans. Louis J. Gallagher (New York: Random House, 1942), 96. I owe this reference to Yang Xiao of Kenyon College, Ohio.

and remember that the majority view has always been that there is more to the world than physics can determine. Maybe the terminally ill are waking up into the world of light,[16] withdrawing their attention from our present dream; we might, on those terms, regard them with awe rather than patronizing or showing indifferent kindness. Some caregivers testify that they have learned from their seemingly incapacitated charges that kindness, courage, and even humor are abiding values.

But just as the currently popular claim that only *persons* are to be respected is contentious, so also is the way we characterize spiritual values as having to do with kindness, courage, humor, and the rest. The spiritual dimensions of healing, as some describe them, have to do with *community* values, understood to involve the companionable virtues. Maybe they are right — but we should remember that other peoples, at other times, have had a lower opinion of *communities*, or else a very different conception of what makes a *good* community. To our predecessors, our own liking for *comfortable* lives would have seemed dishonorable. The emotions and practices that they affirmed and found some sort of spiritual comfort in had to do with honor, courage, or purity. The spiritual dimension of healing, for them, would not have been concerned with kindness but with courage: pain was something to be endured and triumphed over, not to be eliminated (no doubt in part because it was impossible to eliminate such pain). Even cock fights and bear baiting were invested, by our ancestors, with a spiritual value. And even we can be moved by Saint Francis's address to the burning iron used to cauterize his cataracts, in the hope of curing his blindness: moved — but also very disinclined to copy him.

Not all humanistic concern, even of those who would be considered persons, deserves to be called spiritual. When Abishag the Shunammite was brought to cherish and to warm King David, her function was certainly more than that of a warmed brick (1 Kings 1:1–4). No doubt there were ordinarily physiological effects and also mental or emotional ones — but would this count as a spiritual dimension? Perhaps it would, if King David thereby experienced a returning sense of immortal beauty. This too may be a reminder that spirituality — if this is understood to involve acquaintance with what is taken to be divine — has many shapes. King David was probably not practicing the sort of romantic spirituality that De Rougemont ascribed to the medieval troubadours — languishing after a beauty that was deliberately not sought in marriage, without

16. See Henry Vaughan, *Poetry and Selected Prose*, ed. L. C. Martin (London: Oxford University Press, 1963), 318.

trying to consummate desire.[17] But some people have practiced this or similar devices, sometimes in conscious memory of Plato's advice on the uses of erotic love. "If they remain chaste there is no error in their intimacy with the beauty here below, but it is error to fall away into sexual intercourse" (in Plotinus, *Enneads* 3.5 [50].1, 36–37). Would such an erotic element to the healing enterprise be acceptable? Or is that too much for a fallen humanity to risk (and likely to get the therapist disbarred)? When stirring music is played to rouse the martial ardor of a tired or wounded soldiery, this too could be considered spiritual comfort and probably more effective than a chaplain's sermons. Is a community united in martial fervor spiritually healthier than one focused on its several homely comforts? Violence can be invigorating, and agonistic relationships as absorbing as hedonic ones.[18] Our predecessors knew that there were many gods, many moods and modes of conscious being, and knew that all of them were also dangerous. Even the objectifying, distancing eye of Apollo (the god, so to speak, of objective science) is also, in Greek myth, a bringer of pestilence, a destructive lover.[19]

> Highs and peaks say nothing about the worth of a person undergoing them, for they can occur also in psychopaths and criminals, having nothing to do either with creativity or maturity, Maslow's goals. Any textbook of abnormal psychology bears witness to the fact that pathologizing itself can produce peaks: kleptomaniac stealing, pyromaniac barn-burning, sadism, grave desecrations — all can provide ecstatic joys. So can bombing and bayoneting, and so can watching them on television.[20]

The acceptable spiritual dimensions of healing, in brief, depend on our notion of spiritual health: What mode of consciousness, what sort of society, is it that is likeliest to count as an elevation to the divine? Are we to exercise a merely personal choice between them, as though we could ourselves "judge angels"?[21] And is such an elevation strictly desirable?

---

17. Denis de Rougemont, *Passion and Society*, trans. M. Belgion (London: Faber, 1956).

18. The distinction was drawn by Michael R. A. Chance in considering the different styles available to social mammals like ourselves: do we measure ourselves against each other by quarrelling or bond by mutual grooming? See M. R. A. Chance and Donald R. Omark, eds., *Social Fabrics of the Mind* (Hove: Erlbaum Associates, 1988).

19. See my *Civil Peace and Sacred Order* (Oxford: Clarendon, 1990), 160–61.

20. James Hillman, *Re-Visioning Psychology* (New York: Harper Collins, 1975), 66, criticizing what he reckons as Abraham Maslow's "hedonistic philosophy."

21. See 1 Cor. 6:3. Paul's hope (and his consequent advice to the Corinthians not to resort

> Stupid men believe this sort of talk as soon as they hear "you shall be better than all, not only men, but gods" — for there is a great deal of arrogance among men — and the man who was once meek and modest, an ordinary private person, if he hears "you are the son of God, and the others whom you used to admire are not, nor the beings they venerate according to the tradition received from their fathers; but you are better than the heavens without having taken any trouble to become so" — then are other people really going to join in the chorus? (*Enneads* 2.9 [33].9, 53ff.)[22]

Are we at least spiritually healthier by being more aware of the many modes of consciousness, the many stories that we share, the many fantasies we can indulge? Perhaps some *daimones*, intermediate between human beings and God, are truly demons? Platonists like Plotinus, it is supposed, may require us to attempt a sort of union with the One, stripping off all mortal flummery in a "flight of the alone to the Alone." Other religious witnesses have suspected that this is a flight too high: "what does the Lord require of you, but to do justly, and to love mercy, and to walk humbly with your God?" (Mic. 6:8). Maybe pursuit of any mystical union is to think too much of an ideal health, when all that most of us could even *hope* to manage is to relieve particular diseases, disabilities, or sins. And even Plotinus, as I shall suggest, had less in common with such idealists than might be expected. If we cannot reasonably expect full spiritual health, how well can we identify the proper spiritual dimensions of healing? If we cannot be sure what those dimensions are, what hope have we of utilizing spiritual means to heal? If we invoke demons, maybe they will come.

Human beings have devised all kinds of rituals to bring out in themselves different emotions, different attitudes, different ways of perceiving the world. These are significant and should be noticed, but they are not all going to be the same. Not everybody's God — that is, the object of their devotion, the spirit with which they seek to align themselves — is the same as everybody else's. The rituals, the performances, and the texts that we repeat to ourselves are channeled in one direction or another, and if we are going to talk about spiritual dimensions of healing, we must talk about these grand narratives. What is the goal? What is a healthy person? When is an *integrated* person reintegrated back into community? What sort of community are we talking about? Those are questions

---

to Roman law to settle their disputes) rested not on a claim to spiritual superiority but on the presence of the Holy Spirit, made visible (perhaps) in "the gifts of the spirit" (see 1 Cor. 12–13; Gal. 5:22–23).

22. Also see Plotinus, *Enneads*, vol. 2, p. 261, in which A. H. Armstrong suggests a comparison with Irenaeus's protest against the Gnostics in *Against Heresies* 2.30.

that can sometimes be put aside. We can say that there is an immense variety in a pluralistic society, but that we can all get on, more or less, and allow each other to do so, and we can humanistically — if we happen to be in the trade — help people in their particular reintegrations.

But though some commentators hold to something close to that, they also usually back away when faced by certain pictures of humanity and community that they cannot live with (ones animated by militaristic fervor or ethnocentric pride, for example, or else the seemingly self-destructive practices of anorexia).[23] In which case, what are they to do? Is there anything further to say? Is there any sense in which one side is right and the other wrong, or is it going to come down to a matter of brute survival? The Nazis lost, and therefore we do not have to worry about them anymore — though this is plainly false. So the hermeneutical position — according to which we are simply interpreting, telling different stories about what we do and what we are — is likely at some point to encounter some such radical fundamental disagreement, some story we must simply contradict. The less we have reflected on our own ideals, the more astounded and aggrieved we shall be by disagreement.

> The average agnostic of recent times has really had no notion of what he meant by religious liberty and equality. He took his own ethics as self-evident and enforced them; such as decency or the error of the Adamite heresy. Then he was horribly shocked if he heard of anybody else, Moslem or Christian, taking his ethics as self-evident and enforcing them; such as reverence or the error of the Atheist heresy. . . . Medieval men thought that if a social system was founded on a certain idea it must fight for that idea.[24]

Must we then just fight each other because we cannot do anything else? We are telling different stories, and, unfortunately in the end, they are going to be incompatible stories, not simply because they cannot all be *true* but because they demand entirely different lives. Now, that is a very sad situation to be in, but it may of course be true that this is indeed our situation. And if it *is* true, if there is at least *that* truth, we can at least imagine that there might be other truths. In other words, we might start doing the metaphysics and the hard theological and doctrinal graft. "Religion lite" must in the end resort to religion and to metaphysics or else leave us with no recourse but war. Who is right? What is the

---

23. Which would once have been understood as the ascetic practices of likely saints: see Rudolph M. Bell, *Holy Anorexia* (Chicago: University of Chicago Press, 1986).

24. G. K. Chesterton, *St. Francis of Assisi* (London: Hodder & Stoughton, 1996), 144–45.

world? What aspects of healing or life in general give us a clue, which we can reasonably follow up, as to what the truth of things may be? Who is it that can actually "judge angels" (that is, traditional practices and ways of seeing) without being obviously arrogant? People might back away and say, despairingly or complacently, that we have no access to truth. That itself is a metaphysical picture. That itself says we are a certain sort of creature — namely, one incapable of discovering what the truth is — or alternatively that the world is such that there is no true grand narrative. All those are themselves contentious metaphysical positions. So the attempt to reject the idea of a metaphysical resolution itself depends upon having attained a metaphysical resolution (though not one that will do us any good). It is not unreasonable, at least, to ask what metaphysics could accommodate what we wish to be accommodated and guide us, to some extent, in the choices we inevitably make, in the details. We *want* it to be the case that our lives can have some meaning over and above the immediate sensation. We *want* it to be the case that it is possible without extreme bad faith actually to be in community with other creatures in the world and to find out more about that world. We *want* it to be the case that when we find ourselves in various forms of distress — sometimes picked out by our prior metaphysical commitments — we can do something about it. We *want* to rely, sometimes, on our judgment that some practices are wrong, that some ways of seeing are, pejoratively, fantasies. If we want those things to be the case, what sort of universe, what cosmological reality, has it got to be if those wishes have any chance of being satisfied?

The fact that the universe would have to be like that (whatever that is) to satisfy us does not prove the universe is like that (or so it seems to us). But if the universe is *not* like that, then our deepest wants and requirements are not going to be satisfied. In which case, there seems no good reason to continue talking. Accordingly, I shall go on assuming that meaning is possible and that finding out the truth is possible. And so I shall also assume that the universe must be such as to allow us to do this.

Spiritual health requires, at the least, some degree of good faith. If we are to carry on with our lives at any higher level than sensation, we cannot avoid the need for serious thinking about the world, ourselves, and God. Plotinus, as I shall now turn to show, can assist us in this. No doubt there are other spiritual teachers, pagan or otherwise, who can do so too. My preference for working with Plotinus rests partly on historical personal accident and — more significantly — on his abiding presence in the background of so many spiritual and philosophical traditions. Even those who come to disagree with him or with his writings can profit from the discovery that there is something that we may rationally disagree about. But I also hope to show that his proposals are more robust and much less self-serving than much recent spiritual discourse — and that this is a good thing.

Plotinus on Healing

In his treatise *Against the Gnostics* (which was actually the final part of a much larger work upon our duties in the world, distributed by Porphyry into 3.8 [30]; 5.8 [31]; 5.5 [32]; and 2.9 [33] of the *Enneads*), Plotinus mocks sectarian attempts to cure disease by exorcising demons and the use of charms.

> They themselves most of all impair the inviolate purity of the higher powers. . . . For when they write magic chants, intending to address them to those powers, not only to the soul but to those above it as well, what are they doing except making the powers obey the word and follow the lead of people who say spells and charms and conjurations, any one of us who is well skilled in the art of saying precisely the right things in the right ways, songs and cries and aspirated and hissing sounds and everything else which their writings say has magic power in the higher world? . . . When they say they free themselves from diseases, if they meant they did so by temperance and orderly living, they would speak well; but in fact they assume that the diseases are evil spirits, and claim to be able to drive them out by their word; by this claim they might make themselves more impressive in the eyes of the masses, who wonder at the power of magicians, but would not persuade sensible people that diseases do not have their origin in strain or excess or deficiency or decay, and in general in changes which have their origin outside or inside. The cures of diseases make this clear too. With a vigorous motion of the bowels or the giving of a drug the illness goes through the downward passage and out, and it goes out too with bloodletting; and fasting also heals. Does the evil spirit starve, and does the drug make it waste away? . . . If it came into the man without any cause of disease, why is he not always ill? But if there was a cause, what need is there of the spirit to produce the illness? For the cause is sufficient by itself to produce the fever. (*Enneads* 2.9 [33].14)

Augustine, it should be noted, also dismissed magical cures:

> It is one thing to say, "if you drink this plant ground up, your stomach will not hurt," and another to say, "if you hang this plant round your neck, your stomach will not hurt." In the first case the healthful mixture is approved,

in the second the superstitious meaning is condemned. Where there are no incantations and invocations and "characters" it is often doubtful whether the thing that is tied on, or attached in some way for healing the body, works by the force of nature — if so, it can be used freely — or succeeds by some meaningful connection [*significativa quadam obligatione*]: if so, the more effective it seems to be, the more the Christian should be on guard. But where it is not clear why something works, it is the mind-set of the user that matters [*quo animo quisque utatur interest*] in relation to healing or treating bodies, whether in medicine or in agriculture.[25]

The moral was the same, even if the underlying attitude to demons or *daimones* was quite different.[26] Hermeneutical healing, so to call it, dependent on the stories that we tell ourselves and others, is something close to sorcery and to be avoided. As a much later essayist, G. K. Chesterton, observed, "We must see things objectively, as we do a tree; and understand that they exist whether we like them or not. We must not try and turn them into something different by the mere exercise of our minds, as if we were witches."[27] Plotinus's own preferred cures, of course, have not been fashionable in recent years (though there is now some evidence that even bloodletting does occasionally help), but the point here is that he preferred to identify the *causes* of disease by their cures and reckoned illness was only natural.[28] Not that he was himself wholly positive about those cures; according to Porphyry, "he often suffered from a disease of the bowels, but would not submit to an enema, saying that it was unsuitable for an elderly man to undergo this sort of treatment. He refused also to take medicines containing the flesh of wild beasts, giving as his reason that he did not approve of eating the flesh even of domestic animals."[29]

---

25. Augustine, *On Christian Doctrine* 2.110–11, citing the edition and translation of R. P. H. Green (Augustine, *De Doctrina Christiana* [Oxford: Clarendon, 1995]).

26. Marsilio Ficino, in the fifteenth century, also attempted to distinguish *natural* magic from *demonic* magic; see D. P. Walker, *Spiritual and Demonic Magic from Ficino to Campanella* (London: Warburg Institute, 1958), and F. Yates, *Giordano Bruno and the Hermetic Tradition* (London: Routledge & Kegan Paul, 1964).

27. G. K. Chesterton, *Illustrated London News*, November 22, 1913, in *Complete Works*, vol. 29 (San Francisco: Ignatius, 1988), 589, cited by A. DeSilva, ed., *Brave New Family* (San Francisco: Ignatius, 1990), 15. For a further defense of realism, see G. K. Chesterton, *Heretics* (New York: John Lane, 1905), 304–5.

28. Specifically, bloodletting may help in cases of hereditary hemochromatosis, a genetic defect that results in excess accumulation of iron in the pancreas, heart, and liver.

29. Porphyry, *Life of Plotinus* 2, located in Armstrong's edition of Plotinus, *Enneads*, vol. 1, p. 5. On Platonic reasons for vegetarianism, see my "Vegetarianism and the Ethics of Vir-

Porphyry is not an entirely reliable witness about the *motives* of his master; Plotinus was a much more robust and sanguine character than his editor. But the anecdotes perhaps confirm an impression from Plotinus's own writings: he did not merely think that the Gnostic recipes against disease were likely to be ineffective and showed contempt for the powers they professed to control. He did not think their *goals* were good ones. Virtue may, incidentally, be a means to bodily well-being — but those who are truly virtuous care less for bodily well-being than for the god (the thing worth serving) in each and in all of us.[30] "The good man will reduce and gradually extinguish the bodily advantages by neglect, and will put away authority and office. He will take care of his bodily health, but will not wish to be altogether without experience of illness, nor indeed also of pain" (*Enneads* 1.4 [46].14, 19–20).[31] Above all, he will wish to see things truly.

Plotinus did not suppose that we could compel any higher spirits, and when he was invited to accompany a friend to "the temples at the New Moon and the feasts of the gods," he responded that "they ought to come to me, not I to them" (*Enneads* 1.10). The response has been interpreted as an arrogant rejection of those gods, but it is much more likely that he meant that they could not be commanded, that it was for them to descend. We may perhaps create the ambience within which God or the gods can come to us, but we cannot sensibly pursue them. So also Plato distinguished magic and true religion, "in that magic makes every effort to persuade the gods, whereas the truly religious behavior is to leave the gods a free choice, for they know better than we do what is good for us."[32] So how did Plotinus seek to prepare himself for the gods' descent?

> Let there be in the soul a shining imagination of a sphere, having everything within it. . . . Keep this, and apprehend in your mind another, taking away the mass: take away also the places, and the mental picture of matter in yourself,

---

tue," in *Food for Thought: The Debate over Eating Meat*, ed. Steve F. Sapontzis (New York: Prometheus, 2004), 138–51.

30. As Aristotle also said, what matters is *ton theon therapeuein kai theōrein*, "to serve and contemplate the god" (*Eudemian Ethics* 1249b20); see further my "Therapy and Theory Reconstructed," in *Philosophy as Therapeia*, ed. Clare Carlisle and Jonardon Ganeri, Royal Institute of Philosophy Supplement 66 (Cambridge: Cambridge University Press, 2010), 83–102.

31. Note that this was written during the last days of Plotinus's own fatal illness. See also Gillian Clark, "The Health of the Spiritual Athlete," in *Health in Antiquity*, ed. King, 216–29.

32. Fritz Graf, *Magic in the Ancient World* (Cambridge, MA: Harvard University Press, 1999), 27, after Plato, *Laws* 10.903bff. Emma C. Clarke, *Iamblichus' De Mysteriis* (London: Ashgate, 2001), 23–24, points out that Iamblichus, a Neo-Platonist now remembered for preferring theurgic rituals to philosophy, also insisted that the initiative must lie with God.

and do not try to apprehend another sphere smaller in mass than the original one, calling on the god who made that of which you have the mental picture, pray him to come. And may he come, bringing his own universe within him, he who is one and all. (*Enneads* 5.8.9)

Dillon comments:

Here we are being called upon to use our·imagination creatively, to attain to a purely intellectual conception. It is worthwhile, perhaps, to try to perform the exercise as Plotinus prescribes. I have attempted it repeatedly, and the sticking point is always the instruction, once one has conjured up the universe (as a luminous, diaphanous globe, with all its parts distinct and functioning), then to think away the spatiality (*"aphelon ton onkon labe"*) — and not just by shrinking it! It is in fact an excellent spiritual exercise. Calling upon God here is no empty formality. If it is done effectively, it has a quasi-theurgic result: "He may come, bringing his own cosmos, with all the gods that dwell in it — He who is the one God, and all the gods, where each is all, blending into a unity, distinct in powers, but all one god, in virtue of that divine power of many facets." In other words, if you perform the exercise correctly, you will achieve a mystical vision of the whole noetic cosmos. And Plotinus knew what he was talking about.[33]

Dillon, not inappropriately, calls this a spiritual exercise (and testifies to its efficacy), but it is — precisely — not aimed at any material success. Plotinus makes considerable use of guided imagery and even encourages us to think through familiar (or once familiar) myths, like the trials of Dionysus or Prometheus, but not with the goal of restoring bodily health. Like other ancients, he held that "a man has not failed if he fails to win beauty of colors or bodies, or power or office or kingship even, but if he fails to win [the vision of the Good]" (*Enneads* 1.6 [1].7, 34–35), if he has not realized in himself the god on whom he depends, "the god who is in each one of us one and the same" (*Enneads* 6.5.1). The route to that vision of the one original cause and value, Plotinus holds, is by putting aside all merely mortal troubles and demands: "How can this happen? Take away everything!" (*Enneads* 5.3 [49].17, 39). This is not a purely quietist attitude. On the contrary, he urges us to "stand up against the blows of fortune like a great

---

33. John Dillon, "Plotinus and the Transcendental Imagination," in *Religious Imagination*, ed. J. P. Mackey (Edinburgh: Edinburgh University Press, 1986), 55–64, reprinted in John Dillon, *The Golden Chain* (London: Variorum, 1990), 58–59.

trained athlete" (*Enneads* 1.4 [46].8, 25),[34] remembering that "the law says those who fight bravely, not those who pray, are to come safe out of the wars" (*Enneads* 3.2 [47].32, 36–37). But it is also not an attitude that depends upon our successful evasion of pain: witness his blunt reminder that "as far as [the good man's] pains go, when they are very great, he will bear them as long as he can; when they are too much for him, they will bear him off" (*Enneads* 1.4 [46].8, 1ff.).

"And when the pains concern others?" (*Enneads* 1.4 [46].8, 13–14). Decent people nowadays care about others' pains and encourage in themselves an appropriate compassion. It is, therefore, a shock to learn that Plotinus, like the Stoics, thought it weakness to feel for others. "There is evidence for this in the fact that we think it something gained if we do not know about other people's sufferings, and even regard it as a good thing if we die first" (*Enneads* 1.4 [46].8, 14–15).[35] That at least *is* weakness, to be avoided by facing up to what "ordinary nature normally finds terrible" (*Enneads* 1.4 [46].8, 23–24). But modern moralists, and all of us, are more likely to feel that virtue lies in pity and fear,[36] rather than in knowing that "though some natures may not like [such evils], one's own can bear them, not as terrors but as children's bogies" (*Enneads* 1.4 [46].8, 23–24). In the very next treatise that he wrote, he added, "we should be spectators of murders, and all deaths, and takings and sacking of cities, as if they were on the stages of theatres" (*Enneads* 3.2 [47].15, 44–45). Such things are no more than children's games: "one must not take weeping and lamenting as evidence of the presence of evils, for children, too, weep and wail over things that are not evils" (*Enneads* 3.2 [47].15, 61).

> If some boys, who have kept their bodies in good training, but are inferior in soul to their bodily condition because of lack of education, win a wrestle with others who are trained neither in body or soul and grab their food and their dainty clothes, would the affair be anything but a joke? Or would it not be right for even the lawgiver to allow them to suffer this as a penalty for their laziness and luxury? . . . Those who do these things are punished, first by

34. Armstrong translates *athlētēs* as "fighter," but Plotinus is referring to athletic rather than aggressive virtue.

35. Cf. A. D. Nuttall, *A Common Sky: Philosophy and the Literary Imagination* (London: Sussex University Press, 1974), 73ff. Also see Laurence Sterne, *Tristram Shandy* (New York: J. A. Work, 1940), 418.

36. Cf. Augustine, *Confessions* 3.2: "although he that grieves with the grief-stricken is to be commended for his work of charity, yet the man who is fraternally compassionate would prefer to find nothing in others to need his compassion. . . . There is a kind of compassionate sorrow that is good, but there is no kind that we should rejoice to feel."

being wolves and ill-fated men. . . . But the wicked rule by the cowardice of the ruled; for this is just, and the opposite is not. (*Enneads* 3.2 [47].8, 16–21, 26–28, 51–52)

On the one hand, the genuinely virtuous cannot be bullied (or bribed). On the other, such virtuous persons will probably not intervene to prevent such bullying. More than a little alarmingly — to our taste — he is also willing to consider this: "there is no accident in a man's becoming a slave, nor is he taken prisoner in war by chance, nor is outrage done on his body without due cause, but he was once the doer of that which he now suffers; and a man who made away with his mother will be made away with by a son when he has become a woman, and one who has raped a woman will be a woman in order to be raped" (*Enneads* 3.2 [47].13, 11ff.). So though the agent in these cases is wicked (and will suffer in his turn), he has done no real harm — he has indeed, in a sense, done justly. "And if you are wronged, what is there dreadful in that to an immortal?" (*Enneads* 2.9 [33].9, 15–16).

The effort to remember this (however distant from our modern preference) may still be characterized as an attempt at *healing*, though it is the soul rather than the body that is to be healed. It is, literally, *psychotherapy* — but a more robust variety than we now fancy. Plotinus follows Plato in this, as in many other things: our soul may be weighed down and barnacled with vices, and needs to undergo a proper purgation to be healthy again. There is also a role for "exercises to improve our mental grasp . . . an empowering of the soul, just like physical training of our arms and legs" (*Enneads* 4.6 [41].3, 29–30). But these too are only steps along the way. "One must say that this [real] virtue is a kind of intellect and not count in with it the passions which are enslaved and limited by the reason; for these, Plato says, come close to the body, since it is by habits and exercises that they are set in order" (*Enneads* 6.8.6, 22–23). Virtue, that is, is not the same as self-control, nor something that we can be coached or cured into displaying (even though we can perhaps prepare the way by practicing the civic virtues). In effect, it is by grace. Its content is to face up to reality.

When we look outside that on which we depend we do not know that we are one, like faces which are many on the outside but have one head inside. But if someone is able to turn around, either by himself or having the good luck to have his hair pulled by Athena herself, he will see God and himself and the all. . . . He will stop marking himself off from all being and will come to the All without going out anywhere.[37] (*Enneads* 6.5 [23].7, 9–10)

37. The reference is to an episode in the *Iliad*, when Achilles is saved from homicidal rage by Athena's intervention (*Iliad* 1.197–98).

Plotinian Spirituality

So what is a Plotinian spirituality, and why should it concern us? The term is not Plotinus's, of course, though it could be argued that *nous* plays a role very similar to spirit: it is toward one and the same *nous* that all our souls aspire.

> Intellect [*nous*] is our king. But we too are kings when we are in accord with it; we can be in accord with it in two ways, either by having something like its writing written in us like laws, or by being as if filled with it and able to see it and be aware of it as present. (*Enneads* 5.3 [49].3, 46ff.)

The intellect to which he is referring, it must be added, is not the intellectuality of those who are good at reasoning things out, whether in mathematical science or historical inquiry. *Nous* is the immediate grasp of truth, and in seeking for it we are seeking to be joined with truth: to be, truthfully, inspired. Seeking that kingship only, putting aside all other lesser things, freeing ourselves or being freed from the enchantments of the flesh are all notions that our Christian predecessors would have found familiar.

> Your boasting is not a good thing. Do you not know that a little yeast leavens the whole batch of dough? Clean out the old yeast so that you may be a new batch, as you really are unleavened. For our paschal lamb, Christ, has been sacrificed. Therefore, let us celebrate the festival, not with the old yeast, the yeast of malice and evil, but with the unleavened bread of sincerity and truth. (1 Cor. 5:6–8)[38]

Finding such recipes too uncomfortable, we moderns have usually preferred to think that we can have the lesser pleasures, too, and that those who supposed otherwise were unduly negative. We have preferred — as many modern therapists prefer — the model of reintegration to that of purgation; the pursuit of wholeness is sometimes axiomatically identified with the pursuit of health. Those who undertake what they regard as a spiritual path seem to be aiming mainly at being comfortable with themselves, to be reconciled to their own past misdeeds and follies — but not to pay for them. Plotinus's imagery, and Paul's, is purgative: it is necessary to purify ourselves as gold is purified (*Enneads* 1.6 [1].5,

---

38. See also Matt. 18:8: "If your hand or your foot causes you to stumble, cut it off and throw it away; it is better for you to enter life maimed or lame than to have two hands or two feet and to be thrown into the eternal fire."

5off.).[39] It is true that the charge of negativity is one that Plotinus might have recognized: his complaint against the Gnostics — quite apart from their reliance on charms to compel spirits — was that they despised this world. "For over and above need there is in the objects of perception a knowing which brings a not uncivilized pleasure, of the sun and the other heavenly bodies, and the sky and the earth, for instance: for the perception of these is pleasant in itself" (*Enneads* 4.4 [28].22, 39–40). What is to be put aside at a sensual level may still be a proper guide to something better.

So what does aiming for the higher amount to? How are we to ascend?

> It does no good at all to say "Look to God," unless one also teaches how one is to look. . . . In reality it is virtue which goes before us to the goal and, when it comes to exist in the soul along with wisdom, shows God; but God, if you talk about him without true virtue, is only a name. Again, despising the universe and the gods in it and the other noble things is certainly not becoming good. . . . For anyone who feels affection for anything at all shows kindness to all that is akin to the object of his affection, and to the children of the father that he loves. But every soul is a child of That Father. (*Enneads* 2.9 [33].15, 33–16.10)

Every soul, in fact, is Aphrodite, goddess of erotic beauty.

> When it is there [that is, in the intelligible realm] it has the heavenly love, but here love becomes vulgar; for the soul there is the heavenly Aphrodite, but here becomes the vulgar Aphrodite, a kind of whore. And every soul is Aphrodite. . . . The soul then in her natural state is in love with God and wants to be united with him; it is like the noble love of a girl for her noble father.[40] (*Enneads* 6.9 [9].9, 28ff.)

Plotinus's love is not a feeble thing: "these experiences must occur whenever there is contact with any sort of beautiful thing, wonder and a shock of delight and longing and passion and a happy excitement [*ptoēsis meth' hēdonēs*]" (*Enneads* 1.6 [1].4).

---

39. It is not obvious that we can do this for ourselves.

40. In the usual Greek tradition, it is Athena, not Aphrodite, who is "all for the father" (Aeschylus, *Eumenides* 734), and Aphrodite is of an earlier generation of gods, sister to the Titans whom Zeus overthrew.

Intellect [*nous*] also, then, has one power for thinking, by which it looks at the things in itself, and one by which it looks at what transcends it by a direct awareness and reception, by which also before it saw only, and by seeing acquired intellect and is one. And that first one is the contemplation of Intellect in its right mind, and the other is Intellect in love, when it goes out of its mind "drunk with the nectar"; then it falls in love, simplified into happiness by having its fill, and it is better for it to be drunk with a drunkenness like this than to be more respectably sober. (*Enneads* 6.7 [38].35)

We are encouraged, that is, to be "in love," but not with any merely mortal flesh and not with any expectation of return. We are not merely to understand reality, or even to enjoy it, but to be in awe of it. "What does 'really exist' mean? That they exist as beauties" (*Enneads* 1.6 [1].5, 18–19). "Or rather, beautifulness is reality" (*Enneads* 1.6 [1].6, 21).[41] Loving only the source of beauty, we are to lose all lesser things. Loving that, we are to remember who we are: "Even before this coming to be we were there, men who were different, and some of us even gods, pure souls and intellect united with the whole of reality; we were parts of the intelligible, not marked off or cut off but belonging to the whole; and we are not cut off even now" (*Enneads* 6.4 [22].14, 18ff.). To recall ourselves is to cast off that "other man," who has "wound himself round us," so that we here and now have come to be double. Moralists in a related tradition would not, I think, be entirely wrong to note the obvious parallel. "It is now the moment for you to wake from sleep. For salvation is nearer to us now than when we became believers; the night is far gone, the day is near. Let us then lay aside the works of darkness and put on the armor of light" (Rom. 13:11–12).

Paul's metaphors are, of course, significantly different from Plotinus's. Whereas Plotinus urges us to *strip* and so discover our celestial selves, Paul expects instead that the perishable will be *reclothed* with immortality and made over into the likeness of the "last Adam," which is Christ (1 Cor. 15:45).[42] But

---

41. "For this reason being is longed for because it is the same as beauty, and beauty is lovable because it is being" (*Enneads* 5.8 [31].9, 41).

42. The author of the Epistle to the Hebrews, on the other hand, did make use of the stripping motif: "let us also lay aside every weight and the sin that clings so closely, and let us run with perseverance the race that is set before us" (Heb. 12:1). See also Porphyry, *On Abstinence from Eating Animals* (London: Duckworth, 2000), 43 (book 1, paragraph 31): "Let us go stripped, without tunics, to the stadium, to compete in the Olympics of the soul. Stripping off is the starting point, without which the contest will not happen." I have discussed the history and meaning of the metaphor at greater length in "Going Naked into the Shrine: Herbert, Plotinus and the Constructive Metaphor," in *Platonism at the Origins of Modernity:*

both agree that we have something to lose before we manifest that likeness. Later Christians, with whatever careful qualifications, suspected that those who were to be made into that likeness must already, in a sense, be what they are to be, even if they do not yet appear as such. Pagan Neoplatonists, conversely, were not all persuaded by Plotinus that there was a part of us that has never "descended" or fallen at all (*Enneads* 4.8 [6].8). Like Julian of Norwich, he reckoned, we might say, that "in every soul to be saved is a godly will that has never consented to sin."[43] And if it has never descended, never fallen, never sinned, how can it be "cured"?

> But how is the good man affected by magic and drugs? He is incapable of being affected in his soul by enchantment, and his rational part would not be affected, nor would he change his mind; but he would be affected in whatever part of the irrational in the All there is in him, or rather this part would be affected; but he will feel no passionate loves provoked by drugs, if falling in love happens when one soul assents to the affection of the other. But just as the irrational part of him is affected by incantations so he himself by counter-chants and counter-incantations will dissolve the powers on the other side. (*Enneads* 4.4 [28].43)

Those counter-chants and counter-incantations are the arguments that Plotinian philosophers employ to direct their attention where it first belongs, away from practical concerns both personal and public, to the abiding truth (*Enneads* 4.4 [28].43, 19ff.).[44] As Armstrong has written, "philosophical discussion and reflection are not simply means for solving intellectual problems (though they are and must be that). They are also charms for the deliverance of the soul."[45] Rather than careful redescriptions of our condition with a view to getting comfortable with who we are, they are an attempt to cut away delusion and, by

---

Studies on Platonism and Early Modern Philosophy, ed. D. Hedley and S. Hutton (Dordrecht: Springer, 2008), 45–62.

43. Julian of Norwich, *Revelations of Divine Love*, trans. Clifton Wolters (New York: Penguin, 1966), 118.

44. See further my "Charms and Counter-Charms," in *Conceptions of Philosophy*, ed. Anthony O'Hear, Royal Institute of Philosophy Supplement 65 (Cambridge: Cambridge University Press, 2010), 215–31.

45. A. H. Armstrong, "Plotinus," in *Cambridge History of Later Greek and Early Mediaeval Philosophy*, ed. A. H. Armstrong (Cambridge: Cambridge University Press, 1967), 195–271, here 260, after Plotinus, *Enneads* 5.3 [49].17.

separating ourselves from error, from dream and delirium, fantasy, to achieve true permanent community.

"Contemplation alone remains incapable of enchantment because no one who is self-directed is subject to enchantment" (*Enneads* 4.4 [28].44). Magic perhaps works, even at a physical level, thanks to the sympathy that pervades the natural universe and is as accessible to the wicked as the virtuous ("for the wicked draw water from the streams and that which gives does not know itself to what it gives, but only gives" [*Enneads* 4.4 [28].42, 15–16]).[46] Plotinus's disciples apparently believed that he could fend off magical attacks, returning them upon their perpetrator,[47] but it is more likely that he ignored them. Plotinus's spirituality lies in his insistence that our task is to look aside from everything that the users of enchantment most desire. In a sense, it is true that this life here is a play, a costume drama, or a dream. We may hope to get a better (that is, a more responsible) part next time if we manage not to be dragged down this time. We may hope to escape entirely (a thought that modern moralists brand "escapist," uneasily ignoring Tolkien's aphorism that those who most object to escapes are jailers). "Why should a man be scorned, if, finding himself in prison, he tries to get out and go home? Or if, when he cannot do so, he thinks and talks about other topics than jailers and prison-walls? The world outside has not become less real because the prisoner cannot see it."[48]

Plotinus's own belief in reincarnation (however cautious or ironical it may have been) may suggest that he would have sympathized with modern therapists who ask us to take our own "past lives" at least as therapeutic tools.[49] If this life here is only an episode, it must seem sensible to try to recall what other lives we've lived. Even if there are no other lives, it may seem that we can profit from *imagining* what life would have been like for us in other times and places. At the very least, those philosophers who deny even the possibility of such other lives must in effect be saying that I *could not possibly* be anyone but the mortal person who I am — and in that case, how can I engage my moral imagination? Ordinary moral reasoning rests on the possibility of conceiving myself into another's

46. See also Matt. 5:45: Your Father "makes his sun rise on the evil and on the good, and sends rain on the righteous and on the unrighteous."

47. *Life of Plotinus* 10, located in Armstrong's edition of Plotinus, *Enneads*, vol. 1, p. 33.

48. J. R. R. Tolkien, "On Fairy Stories," in *Tree and Leaf; Smith of Wooton Major; The Homecoming of Beorhtnoth Beorhthelm's Son* (London: Unwin, 1975), 61.

49. See Roger J. Woolger, *Other Lives, Other Selves: A Jungian Psychotherapist Discovers Past Lives* (New York: Doubleday, 1987), and Brian L. Weiss, *Through Time into Healing: How Past Life Regression Therapy Can Heal Mind, Body and Soul* (London: Piatkus, 1992).

place and so creates at least the *imaginative* possibility of other lives.[50] When we recall that we might play other parts and that the natures we now wear are only borrowed glories, it is possible to greet all others as the spiritual equals — or superiors — they are. Because I know I *might have been* a tramp, a leper, or a lord (or else a dog, a star, or a spider — or even a rapist or a rape victim), I know that the ones who variously *are* those things (who wear those natures) are greater than the parts they play. But though Plotinian cosmology permits us to have many lives, it does not follow that he wants us to *remember* them, still less to fantasize about them.[51] On the contrary, we should not be taking such passing episodes seriously enough to recall them afterward: "the more [the soul] presses on towards the heights the more it will forget, unless perhaps all its life, even here below, has been such that its memories are only of higher things; since here too it is best to be detached from human concerns, and so necessarily from human memories" (*Enneads* 4.3 [27].32, 12ff.).

It is no part of a Plotinian philosopher's task to insist on bodily health, and even the health of the soul — which is conceived as something that needs exercises and purgations — is in the end irrelevant. Even in the bull of Phalaris, even in the utmost agony, "there is another which, even while it is compelled to accompany that which suffers pain, remains in its own company and will not fall short of the vision of the universal good" (*Enneads* 1.4 [46].13, 6ff.). Neither the health of the body nor the health of the soul resides in being made whole, nor even in being reconciled with our immediate community. After all, even if it is true that we still have some connection with an unfallen spirit, it is also true that we are here because we fell; our deepest self may not be our *best* self, as moderns usually propose. Finding out what we are really like may not be quite so comforting a thing. What matters is that we be purged and that we keep our eye on God. This is not, after all, a retreat from life but its discovery.

> It is like a choral dance: in the order of its singing the choir keeps round its leader but may sometimes turn away so that he is out of their sight, but when it turns back to him it sings beautifully and is truly with him; so we are always around him — and if we were not, we should be totally dissolved and

50. See G. Madell, *The Idea of the Self* (Edinburgh: Edinburgh University Press, 1981).

51. It is a standard trope among those wishing to discredit reincarnationist claims that people remember only being royalty or the like. Actually, this is simply untrue (see, for example, Ian Stevenson, *Twenty Cases Suggestive of Reincarnation* [Charlottesville: University of Virginia Press, 1988]), but it would hardly be surprising that they remember *memorable* lives. The Plotinian objection to the attempt is not that they are mistaken but that harping on such things does us no good.

no longer exist — but not always turned towards him; but when we do look to him, then we are at our goal and at rest and do not sing out of tune as we truly dance our god-inspired dance around him.[52] (*Enneads* 6.9 [9].8, 38ff.)

We fell (or we are fallen creatures) because we turned aside from that, each hoping to have things our way.[53] Augustine offers the same moral. There is a difference between public ritual, dedicated to the service of the One God, and private rituals (sorcerous acts) that serve the self-interest of the sorcerer or divert attention away from greater goods.[54] The model that Augustine chiefly uses for magic is that it rests upon an implicit compact with demons, who assuredly do not have our good at heart.[55] Plotinus's complaint against the Gnostics was that they did not treat the gods with proper respect, but he too could draw a line between those gods, *daimones*, and heroes whose eyes were turned toward the One and those who were themselves obsessed with comfort, bodily health, or public wealth. Pagan and Christian alike were sure that spiritual healing lay in putting aside those things that seem at first to matter most to us and turning entirely toward the One, toward what he identifies as "the power of [or in] all things" (*Enneads* 3.8.10).[56]

The full implications of that turn, and what a genuine Plotinian saint would be, would require a much longer exposition.[57] There would certainly be theoretical and practical difficulties to be resolved — and that is what the tradition of theological speculation in Christendom, Judaism, and Islam, as well as the parallel traditions of Hindu and Buddhist thought, have been engaged upon. There are many different ways of developing Plotinian philosophy, as the dif-

52. See also *Enneads* 2.2 [14].2, 15–16: "since [the soul] cannot go to [God], it goes round him." Armstrong translates *koryphaion* as "conductor," but the reference is much more likely to be to the lead dancer.

53. See *Enneads* 4.8 [6].4, 11–12: "As if they were tired of being together, they each go to their own."

54. Plato made the same distinction in *Laws* 10.909dff. As Benjamin Jowett translates it: "there should be one law, which will make men in general less liable to transgress in word or deed, and less foolish, because they will not be allowed to practise religious rites contrary to law. And let this be the simple form of the law: — No man shall have sacred rites in a private house."

55. See R. A. Markus, *Signs and Meanings: World and Text in Ancient Christianity* (Liverpool: Liverpool University Press, 1996), 125–46.

56. See Eric D. Perl, "The Power of All Things," *American Catholic Philosophical Quarterly* 71 (1997): 301–13.

57. Which I have partly attempted in *Plotinus: Myth, Metaphor, and Philosophical Practice* (Chicago: University of Chicago Press, 2016).

ferences between his pagan, Christian, Jewish, and Islamic heirs make clear. The moral for my present examination of the spiritual dimensions of healing must be, at least, that our notions of spiritual health are problematic, open to challenge from recognizably honest and honorable thinkers. If Plotinus was even approximately correct (and generations of his heirs have held that he was), then spiritual health lies in the recognition of reality both as something Other than our ordinary delirium and as something that sustains and enriches even that delirium. Not all spirits tell the truth, but that they speak at all may give us a clue to what the truth may be — and that it is to be preferred to any stories that we merely tell ourselves.

And to conclude with a return to the spooky story that identifies this as a merely *virtual* reality: we have dreamt ourselves into this predicament and must recall ourselves. But it need not follow that we should wake entirely or wholly ignore the world of present experience. On the contrary, that would be to refuse the challenge. We have set ourselves, or have been set, to cope with horrors and absurdities and magic charms. Our health lies in engaging with that challenge: doing justly, loving mercy, and walking humbly with our God. By Plotinus's account, as well as Saint John's, that God is Love — but what either of them meant by this requires a lifetime's work.[58]

---

58. *Enneads* 6.8 [39].15 (*erōs*); see 1 John 4:8 (*agapē*). The fact that the Greek words are different does not mean that the concept is not the same — any more than the fact that there is only one *English* word means that the concepts are not different.

Part Four

Anthropological and Pastoral Perspectives

9

Contemporary Healing in Anthropological Perspective

Thomas J. Csordas

Anthropology is best equipped to bring two things to an interdisciplinary discussion of healing. One is an approach that circumvents theological commitment for the sake of emphasizing the practices and effects of healing, while recognizing that others may observe theological implications in these very practices and effects. The other is to add a comparative perspective to our deliberations, posing the question of how to understand experience across healing traditions originating in radically different cultural milieus. This is, first, in effect a phenomenological comparison insofar as the phenomena of healing must be bracketed from attributions about their source and efficacy, and, second, the physical, moral, and spiritual antecedents and consequences of healing must be appreciated in the specificity of their social milieu.[1] My examples will be Catholic Charismatic spiritual healing among the

---

1. For further discussion of the methodology I employ in this chapter, see my book, *The Sacred Self: A Cultural Phenomenology of Charismatic Healing* (Berkeley: University of California Press, 1994), especially the preface and chapter 1. In the book, I make a similar claim to blend a phenomenological account of the self (grounded in the work of Merleau-Ponty and Bourdieu) with first-person interpretive accounts of healing experience. I claim that "there is an experiential specificity of effect in religious healing — that transformative meaning dwells, to borrow a phrase from the poet William Blake, in the 'minute particulars' of human existence taken up in the healing process" (p. 3). In order to examine this experiential specificity, I claim in *The Sacred Self* that we must "work out our insights in the empirical thickness of healers' and supplicants' experience, specifying the transformation

North American middle classes and Navajo Indian spiritual healing as practiced in the southwestern United States.

In what manner do participants in religious healing become existentially engaged in the healing process? Many of our accounts of performance in ritual healing analyze the sequence of action and the organization of text, but rarely do they investigate the phenomenology of healing and being healed. The shaman's formal narration of a journey to the realm of spirits is taken as data, but he or she is rarely questioned about the qualities of that realm and what it is like to move about in it. The patient is even less a presence, frequently treated as a mere spectator rather than someone who is caught up in an experience that may be more or less immediate and vivid and that he or she may not understand. Yet the nature of this engagement would appear to be critical to the efficacy of religious healing.

This problem was suggested to me by observing the occurrence of imagery in patients of Navajo medicine men and Catholic Charismatic healers. Among the former, it was possible retrospectively to elicit detailed accounts of imagery sequences that occurred in healing sessions. These sequences in many cases amounted to elaborate imaginal performances including the patient, significant others, and deities. Yet the details of these performances were not only invisible in the healing sessions but also were not necessarily narrated to the healer afterward.

In this chapter, I will describe episodes from the healing process undergone by two patients, with the goal of providing material for discussion of cultural differences in the experience of healing. Following each presentation, I will analyze that patient's experience in terms of what I have called the rhetorical model of a therapeutic process. This is a descriptive model of performative and persuasive dimensions of spiritual healing, intended to be of use across different cultures and systems of healing. Briefly stated, the four components of the model of therapeutic process include the following:

1. The *disposition* of supplicants, both in the psychological sense of their prevailing mood or tendency for engagement in ritual performance and

---

of suffering and distress as the transformation of self" (p. 15) where the self is understood as an interactive locus between the world and one's conscious constitution of the world. This leads me to adopt a method that "not only describes Charismatic healing practices in cultural context, but realizes that a full account includes the Charismatics' interpretation of their own practices" (p. xi).

in the physical sense of how they are disposed vis-à-vis the social networks and symbolic resources of the religious community.

2. The *experience of the sacred*, taking into account the religious formulation of the human condition in relation to the divine, the repertoire of ritual elements that constitute legitimate manifestations of divine power, and variations in individual capacities for experience of the sacred that may influence the course of the therapeutic process.

3. The *elaboration of alternatives* or possibilities that exist within the "assumptive world" of the afflicted.[2] Healing systems may formulate these alternatives in terms of a variety of metaphors and may use ritual or pragmatic means that encourage either activity or passivity, but the possibilities must be perceived as real and realistic.

4. The *actualization of change*, including what counts as change as well as the degree to which that change is regarded as significant by participants. This may occur in an incremental and open-ended fashion, without definitive outcome.

Catholic Charismatic Healing

The Catholic Charismatic Renewal began in 1967 among junior faculty and graduate students at Catholic universities, who in a spirit of enthusiastic communitarianism adopted the principal ritual features of Pentecostalism, including baptism in the Holy Spirit, speaking in tongues, and laying on of hands for ritual healing. The movement quickly expanded beyond the campuses into Catholic parishes, religious orders, and abroad. In the United States, active membership reached a peak of over 600,000 in 1976, whereupon it declined to just under 200,000 by the end of the 1980s. Participants are organized into parochial prayer groups headed by pastoral teams of lay and religious leaders, and highly structured intentional groupings called covenant communities headed by coordinators. A substantial degree of uniformity in ideology and ritual practice has been maintained by an extensive literature of books, pamphlets, and audiocassettes, as well as a structure of regional, national, and international service committees.

There are three major genres of Charismatic ritual healing, corresponding to a cultural conception of the person as a tripartite composite of body, mind,

2. See Jerome Frank and Julia Frank, *Persuasion and Healing*, 3rd ed. (Baltimore: Johns Hopkins University Press, 1993).

and spirit. Physical healing is addressed to medical problems, inner healing or healing of memories for emotional or psychological problems, and deliverance to affliction by evil spirits. Performative acts in healing are discrete gestures or verbal formulae construed primarily as acts of empowerment, protection, revelation, and deliverance. Among others, they include the laying on of hands, speaking in tongues, use of Catholic sacramentals, soaking prayer (intense and lengthy sessions in which a patient is "saturated" with prayer), calling down the blood of the Lamb (invocation of the redemptive power of the blood shed by the crucified Christ), word of knowledge (divine revelation), and binding of spirits (ritual command preventing demon disruption of the interpersonal milieu). Finally, the rhetoric of ritual performance is undergirded by an elaborate terminology that designates ideal forms of interpersonal relation, collective organization, personal qualities, and activities in service to the divine plan. On the negative side, a well-developed demonology recapitulates in mirror image virtually every positive item in this terminology.

The following is an account of imaginal performance that occurred in sessions in which the ritual genre enacted is the healing of memories. These sessions are private events with one patient and either one or two healers. The patient sits on a chair, and the healer either sits facing the patient or stands alongside, laying on hands. Periods of conversation — in which the healer asks questions, gives advice, or counsels the patient — alternate with periods of prayer. I was allowed to be present and to audio record healing sessions. Immediately following each session, I used a standardized set of questions to elicit an experiential commentary from the patient. On a separate occasion, I conducted a three-part interview with patients individually, which included questions about their life history, questions on the nature and extent of their participation in the Charismatic movement, and two standard instruments used for psychiatric diagnosis in research settings.

The Man with the German General Within

The healing team of two was led by a Catholic woman aged thirty-eight. She had been involved in the Charismatic Renewal for ten years, beginning with an episode in which she experienced healing prayer in the aftermath of an automobile accident. She worked full-time in a Charismatic counseling center, the staff of which included both psychotherapists and specialists in inner healing. Her own training included a master's degree in counseling, two years apprenticeship in inner-healing prayer, and certification as a spiritual director in the Ignatian method. Her other influences included bioenergetics and dysfunctional-family/

addictive-behavior approaches, making her perhaps the most eclectic healer in our project. She was assisted in her work with this particular male patient by a male inner healer, following the precept that one-on-one healing prayer should not be conducted with participants of opposite sexes.

The patient was a thirty-seven-year-old married man with three children, a college graduate employed in a managerial position. He had participated in the Episcopalian Charismatic Renewal, where he met his wife and participated in an intentional community. However, they were no longer active and reported worshiping now "in a different way," not having prayed in tongues for some time. He defined his principal problem as stress derived from a long-standing self-image that demanded high levels of accomplishment. He felt that guilt and insecurity about inadequate achievement caused diminished enjoyment and a partial "paralysis," in the sense of making it more difficult and time-consuming to achieve particular goals. His preoccupation with accomplishment had created a strain on marital intimacy, in that his wife "didn't feel like she had access to me or wasn't able to have the relationship she wanted to." He reported having had problems with overeating and with preulcerative stomach symptoms. Our diagnostic interview revealed a single episode of alternating mania and depression in college, a simple phobia of heights, and a period of dysthymia and generalized anxiety disorder immediately preceding his recourse to healing. He had encountered the principal healer at a stress management workshop in which she integrated body-relaxation techniques and inner-healing prayer. Weekly counseling and inner-healing prayer had been ongoing for a year and a half when he participated in our project, at which time he felt that he had made progress in a process of healing that he explicitly equated with spiritual growth.

In each session, the female healer took the lead in counseling and "grounding," a bioenergetics technique in which the patient bends over at the waist, breathes deeply, and becomes attentive to embodied imagery, muscular tensions, or sensations. The male healer took the lead in subsequent prayer and imagery processes, during parts of which all three held hands and during other parts of which one or both healers laid hands on the patient. The following is the most significant event the patient selected from the first of five sessions I followed with him. The event occurs in two parts. The first begins with a memory brought forward by the patient of an incident from his high-school years, in which his mother became angry upon discovering that he had arranged an overachieving and "superhuman" academic and athletic schedule that left no moment unaccounted for. The principal healer suggested that this memory be taken into the grounding exercise, and as they began she instructed him, when he straightened his posture, to do the following:

Healer: . . . imagine an image of that person who has insisted that schedule, and a lot of other things in your life that have been superhuman. When you see him, focus on that person's posture and clothing, language and breathing, and see if the spirit inspires you with verbal knowledge of what that person would say. When you're ready, step one step to either side, and take on the person's posture, breathing style, and language, and we'll meet him as you open your eyes when you're ready. (pause)

Suppliant: Very straight, really precise.

H: OK, accentuate everything about him. His face?

S: Rigid.

H: Knees — how are they held?

S: Locked.

H: Lock them and accentuate, and before you talk, what is my body experiencing that tells me about the way I hold in this personality, and we're going to talk to you. OK? . . . "Hello."

S: H'lo. (Using deeper voice)

H: You look rather uh, anxious.

S: No.

H: Under stress. . . .

S: Nope.

H: What's going on in your life?

S: Just trying to get things done.

H: It appears that you asked S to put together this schedule.

S: Yes, it'd be good for him — make him feel good about himself — best thing for him.

H: I'm not really sure that's what S thinks.

S: I think he knows it'll make him — and if he wants to accomplish these things, that's the way to do it.

H: Would you be willing to give us some insight — talk to S about why it's a good idea?

S: Mm-hmm. Discipline is the only way to accomplish anything. If you don't put aside the things you want to do at the moment, then you'll never accomplish anything that you want to accomplish in the long run. It's — life isn't really made for fun; it's really made for accomplishment, [and] satisfaction in that accomplishment. You always strive for the future. . . .

H: You just close your eyes, see what your body's feeling as you relax your hand, relax your breathing, drop your shoulders, drop your head, move back into grounding gently.

S: (loud exhale, both breathe audibly)

H: Just let go of whatever you contained in the last few minutes, breathing it out. Let's start to modulate some of this. When you're ready, gently come up. (S continues audible breathing.) How are you feeling?

S: (returns to normal voice) Relaxed. Very relaxed after that. That was an extreme kind of physical and emotional tension that I'm not completely familiar with. A little shocked at the intensity of the philosophy that's there. I recognized it as something that I've internalized. The goal setting, that it's there or bust.

H: Listen to your language, in terms of the body — bust.

S: I felt — I'm thinking that it's difficult for me to deal with that strength of personality, of — more relaxed part of me would have a hard time being protected against that side of me, because it's so powerful, and has the strength and determination.

H: Two of your favorite statements — did you hear them?

S: One about discipline, and that accomplishment's more important than play.

H: And the other thing that really caught me was "live for tomorrow" — plan for the future, so when you think of the powerlessness of that figure, how does your life live out those three scripts, and move with being obedient to that subpersonality as opposed to being true to yourself.

The patient in this imaginal performance reenacts his memory not by entering a particular situation but by entering, as it were, its underlying motivation. In this episode, the patient, by means of embodied role-playing in what is likely a state of light hypnosis, identifies a controlling "subpersonality." Here embodied imagery is enacted in a transformation of postural model, including vocal posture, as he responds to the healer in a deeper-than-usual voice. Following some additional discussion, the session turns to prayer:

H: Breathe in and breathe out. Breathe in the tranquility of Christ . . . to hear Jesus speak. To feel Jesus touch. In the name of the Father, the Son, and Holy Spirit. You have revealed to us a new person, a new subperson within S. . . . Lord Jesus, we ask for the strength and patience to embrace this new subperson, befriend him, maybe. To begin to look at those good things about him, that has made S successful, and yet has those qualities that tries to overpower him and take away his freedom. Jesus, we ask that you journey with S to meet this person face-to-face, to begin to dialogue with that person — what he wants, what he wants to do within S, and who gives him that authority. Let S ask those questions and let this person respond (pause). . . . Jesus, relax S, sharpen his mind to use this person in the way you want him to, (whispering) befriend him, Lord Jesus. Let that person that is so rigid with you [i.e., in his relation to the deity] know that he is loved also. . . . We just image inside your light — your radiant light moving through S. We see this prayer finding its way to that space, where that controller is hidden, and we see this prayer like a blanket of safety and love, surrounding and quieting him, putting him in his rightful place before you, Jesus, even while we breathe gently, we imagine that controller responding to this prayer by beginning to feel his feelings as we see that part of time that has been lost in an isolated controller, being made open by this prayer; open to his feelings, open to S the essence of who S is. We praise you, Jesus. . . . Just be with your feelings now, S.

[S breathes once audibly, then pause — movement]

S: The question [to the controller in imaginal performance] is "why are you so strong?" and the response [is he's] just following my orders. "If he wants to be different, he just has to tell me. Show me what you want — how you want to relate." We prayed some more, and it was quiet a while. Then we [the controller and the patient] were at a very peaceful spot — a garden with flowers around us. He and I were there together relaxing. He was relaxed, saying [he doesn't] mind this. This is fine, if you want to live this way — no problem. It really wasn't his choice. So I feel the door opened up to dialogue there. . . . He was made controller, but I need to change that name.

H: Exactly. So you can dialogue with him. You [earlier] called him a ge-stapo type. What's all that about?

S: I think it was in the 50s and early 60s when I grew up, you got a lot of prejudice on TV about the Germans, and I just finished reading *The Secret of Santa Vittoria*, and that's probably the reason.

H: In that book, what did the Germans represent?

S: They ruin their fun. The people had to operate underground to avoid the Germans.

To begin describing the elements we have identified as critical to an understanding of therapeutic process in ritual healing, the disposition of this patient was certainly positive. He was both knowledgeable and committed to the process. At the same time, he had a well-developed sense of the intersection between therapy aimed at treating emotion and resolving personality issues, on the one hand, and healing aimed at encountering divinity and fostering spiritual growth, on the other. That he shared this sense with the healers is critical to the nature of engagement in therapeutic process.

With respect to the element of therapeutic process we have called *encounter with the sacred*, it is of note that this sequence of imaginal performance occurs during inner-healing prayer rather than in the bioenergetics grounding exercise. However, while the divine presence is vividly invoked in the prayer, it appears in embodied imagery not as an actor — the figure of Jesus or the Virgin Mary, for example — but as the peaceful setting of a garden where the patient interacts with the controller within himself. The encounter with the sacred takes the form of bodily image and experience on multiple levels. In repeated sessions (not all summarized here), the patient experiences muscular tension in a variety of body parts; in the grounding exercise, he adopts the postural model of — and thereby incarnates — the controlling subpersonality; and in prayer he walks and talks with the controller in a peaceful garden. A final instance of embodied imagery in this process is contributed not by the patient but by the assistant healer. In one session, he reported a vision of Jesus with a child and three other people — the patient and the masculine and feminine aspects of his being. The three "ministered" to the child, and Jesus "merged" the three figures into one.

Throughout the process, the elaboration of alternatives occurs as a series of embodied oppositions. These include tension/relaxation, control/spontaneity, insecurity/intimacy, and masculine/feminine. This in itself corresponds to the rather rigid either-or mentality he expresses, insofar as the alternatives are not formulated as a series of possible choices or as the opening of a new but indeterminate horizon signifying a transformed vision of personal and spiritual reality.

Finally, with respect to the actualization of change, in his experiential commentary, the patient discusses the beginning of reconciliation with the controlling aspect of himself:

> What I was doing was letting myself go so that that part of my personality could come through completely. . . . I felt very relaxed. . . . I was aware of feeling slightly ridiculous and had to not let that emerge. . . . And [then] just really felt, physically, the tension, and I was aware of the kind of physically destructive tension that kind of personality could cause in my body — the stress on my stomach, tension like high-blood-pressure tension, holding

back. And stress, the kind you read about that causes heart disease . . . [but what the imaginal personality] wanted to express was a very externalized facade of discipline, excellence, accomplishment . . . [the experience] helps me become aware of when that kind of stress is going on and how I can control it. It helps me separate out, "OK, now that's what's clicking in — is it really appropriate?" But it's a better sense of making those choices myself rather than having it be an automatic, habitual kind of response. I swim for exercise and health, but also swim for pleasure at my lunch hour, for relaxation. Yet many times, it becomes duty, work, and that kind of discipline taking the joy out of it, the relaxation out of it. Because you *have* to do it. You have to do it *well*. . . . [The imaginal figure represents] places when it's there and doesn't have to be there. It's not that it's discipline but, oh, pressure. Compulsive. . . . The fact that that got isolated — coupled together with the prayer at the end where I was able to then realize that I could be friends or use this part of the personality as a help rather than a hindrance — was the most significant thing. That discipline side of my personality is something that really wants to be on my side. It doesn't really want to fight against me. I think I will find myself with less tension because an awful lot of the stress that I feel is brought on by the internal conflict of this disciplinarian or this controller.

The patient comes to realize not only that his need to be in control controls him but also that he is the one who, by his own choice, set up the controller in the first place. Particularly in the reference to swimming, it is evident that control is understood not only as overachievement but also as the inhibition of spontaneity. In subsequent sessions, he identified a childhood longing for freedom in the face of external controls imposed by teachers and his father. He also identified, as a defense against an insecurity that was a consequence of these controls, the overdevelopment of a sense of discipline that was "not external but feels external." Finally, he discovered a sense of being existentially "lost" between self-indulgence (overeating) and discipline (overwork) and was instructed by the healer to cultivate freedom through his relation to the deity in that in-between space. The psychocultural theme of intimacy is tied into this complex, as it becomes evident that the patient seeks intimacy through making others dependent on his ability to control and "take care of everything." An awareness of maintaining habitual tension in the genital area, without which he felt his body would "collapse or fall apart," is linked to alienation from his masculinity. In the therapeutic logic developed by the healer, his masculinity is the same controller who, if "befriended," will then make way for integration of masculine and feminine sides of his personality and the possibility of true intimacy.

Traditional Navajo Healing

The Navajo, or *Diné* in their own language, number more than two hundred thousand and live in the southwestern United States on the largest Indian reservation in the United States. Their society is traditionally organized around matrilineal clans, and today people make their living through a combination of herding and agriculture, supplemented where possible by wage labor in areas such as mining, railroad work, or government. The Navajo are by no means wealthy, but their broad base of land and resources, along with a viable language and strong efforts to maintain Navajo culture and identity, allow them to preserve a sense of true nationhood. Most important to our interest here, however, is that Navajo religious ceremonies — save for those marking key moments of a person's life cycle, such as birth, puberty, marriage, and death — are almost invariably concerned with the health and well-being of a patient. In traditional Navajo ceremonies, a *hataali*, or chanter, sings long prayers that in minute detail recount and reorder the elements of life, situating the patient in a position of renewed strength and awareness of a unique place in the world.

Traditional healing is predicated on what might be called a *philosophy of obstacles*. Nothing happens without a reason, and the reason for misfortune is encountering an obstacle. Obstacles are identified not only as causes of illness but occur everywhere in life; growing sleepy at one's desk is an example. The problems we encounter are already there before we encounter them. As one chanter said, "It's like we walk into a room and among the problems, where we proceed to get stuck. We must separate them all like strands, make our way through them [makes a gesture like parting bushes in front of himself]." The therapeutic principle of traditional healing is *didactic*. There are multiple techniques available to the healer, and contrary to much of what is understood about ritual healing, they are not ritual manipulations that the patient merely observes as spectator. Instead, they are methods of engaging the patient in the therapeutic process, guiding thought toward the goal of understanding.

Traditional Navajo healing, in addition to formal diagnostic or divinatory techniques, includes a substantial number of named chants that may be performed in abbreviated versions of several hours or full-length versions that last nine days and nights. Each chant is composed of a series of songs that often allow variation to suit the needs of a particular patient, as well as a number of important ceremonial objects and manipulations of these objects (for example, a wedding basket, *jish* or medicine bundle, prayer sticks, corn pollen, water, sacred stones, buckskin) and, finally, carefully constructed sand-paintings with important mythical and cosmological meanings upon which patients are required to sit. The common technique of having the patient repeat lines of the long chants after the chanter has an engaging effect, especially, as one Navajo participant said, when the chant "speeds up into second gear" and one is carried along. As another noted, the proceedings are "ritualistic" only to one who does not understand the Navajo language. One who does understand experiences the contextualization of life experience within a cosmological and physical "home," the Navajo land, and people. The case that follows has to do with the Lightning Way, one of the most important among Navajo ceremonials.[3]

The Man Who Was Struck by Lightning

Jesse is a sixty-nine-year-old retired widower who lives in his own home, sparsely decorated with an old Chevrolet calendar and a velour Christ on the wall. His house is in proximity to those of two of his sisters and their families, on a large piece of traditional family land where he was born and raised. Among the homes and outbuildings is one traditional Navajo house or "hogan," which is used primarily for ceremonial purposes. The family also has a farm nearby, and Jesse's farm work is very important to him. He is a jovial and talkative man, who laughs easily and often, and seems always to have a smile on his face. Though he does not appear particularly reverential or philosophical, he is earnest-appearing and focused, an elder who still has vigorous strength. He speaks primarily in Navajo, and our interviews were in the Navajo language, assisted by an interpreter.

Six of Jesse's eleven siblings are still alive. Family relations seem very important to him, and he said, "Our ceremonial tradition is to love each other." His childhood was "OK," without too much hardship, though his parents were strict and gave the children chores to do. He indicated obliquely that his father was fairly abusive and authoritarian, though his father ended up being his "drinking buddy" during his late teens and early twenties when they worked on the railroad together. Jesse went to day school briefly but said that all they did was pick up trash and, if they didn't pick up enough, they would be whipped. After leaving school, he held many different jobs, including local and migrant farm work, making adobe bricks, railroad work, water-line construction, and a short stint of three to four months mining uranium. He reported having had twelve wives, though most of these were short-term, and he has only four children by the two women to whom he had been officially married. His most recent wife passed away just two months before our interviews. Jesse seems to have cared

3. See Thomas J. Csordas, *Body/Meaning/Healing* (New York: Palgrave, 2002).

for her deeply but said that they did talk of divorce. He said she wanted to leave, partly because she believed that an abundance of "skinwalkers" (sorcerers) were around their home and that witches had planted bundles there as well.

Jesse traces the root of his problems to a traditional Lightning Way ceremony in 1957, when he was around thirty years old. The ceremony was being given for a patient who was himself a Lightning Way singer. During a break in the ceremony, the hogan (traditional Navajo one-room dwelling) was struck by lightning, and a blue flame came down into the hogan through the smoke hole in the roof. Two of the eight people in the hogan were killed, including Jesse's father. "He was just asleep, wrapped in or curled in his blankets. There was another man laying over here . . . lying sideways, and he was thrown up and was ripped down the middle. My father was laying there, and the lightning went through him completely. There were two." Of the two medicine men present, one was lying down and was not injured. The patient was out of the hogan at the time and was uninjured also. Besides the two killed, another man was hit by lightning, but it struck only his leg and he survived. Jesse was thrown unconscious against the wall and went out cold, lying in the doorway. During the time he was unconscious, he saw himself from above the hogan, out of his body.

Jesse and several other members of his family awoke with a jagged, lightning-shaped print across their chests. Two of his sisters who had not been attending the ceremony went into the hogan to help, thus also becoming exposed to the effects of lightning. Following the incident, and before being fully recovered, Jesse had sex with his wife. She died less than a year later. Jesse subsequently learned of his mistake and realized that he had caused her death. Jesse sees much of what has subsequently occurred in his life as being traceable to this event. Indeed, it was an enduring trauma for the entire family, all the more so because of the spiritual danger and ritual power associated in Navajo religion with lightning and ceremonies associated with lightning. Nevertheless, he felt that his contact with lightning was a kind of initiation and that having escaped injury he was "accepted by lightning," thus suggesting a kind of permanent affinity for this powerful force. Having survived while a medicine man had perished may have left him with powerfully divergent messages of his own spiritual strength, combined with a sense of isolation or even alienation from other people in his life. Stated in other terms, it may be describable as the combination of a post-traumatic stress response with the intensification of feelings associated with the violation of strong social conventions.

Jesse reported having had previous ceremonies done for the problem, but these were minor chants that he thought to have failed in part because "the chanters do not do a good, complete job. . . . Nowadays it's all done in haste, right after you make the payment." It is important that something as catastrophic as the lightning strike that killed Jesse's father had never been addressed with a major ceremony. Nevertheless, as is often the case, Jesse said that his symptoms didn't start until much later (fifteen to twenty years), because when he was young, he was "strong in body." In the Navajo view, these delayed effects could have been forestalled if the original chanter had taken steps to correct the situation — including a cooling rite, herbal rinsing rites for the people in the hogan, and construction of a separate shelter in which offerings and a blessing could have been made. These steps were never taken.

At the time he finally contracted a chanter to perform a Lightning Way ceremony (traditionally to remove effects of exposure to lightning), Jesse reported a number of symptoms — including heartburn, aches in his bones and joints, blurred vision, lower-back and leg pain, and dizziness. Plans were also made to integrate elements of another ceremony known as an Evil Way (traditionally to remove effects of exposure to the dead), which Jesse needed following the recent death of his second wife. "The wife that passed away," he told us, "I had to help her through her illness, for about nine years, thereabouts. Because of that, they tell me I'm affected by the Evil Way to a great extent." He said the main symptoms of this were a kind of nervousness, his "mental thinking" gone "astray." At one point, he told us that he often has a lot of trouble when he's inside a large crowded place like a department store: "My heart starts to race and causes me to breathe hard. I feel like I'm stumbling along the aisles, I'm afraid of running into something. You might black out and run head-on into something," he said. In addition, events in his family's life had recently become stressful, as some of his grandchildren had gotten in trouble and several family members had had health difficulties. Our clinical diagnostic interview suggested that he met criteria for dysthymic disorder, though since he appears to have been deeply affected by the wear and tear and worry of having to take care of his terminally ill wife, it is likely that this can be understood as due to the stress of bereavement following his wife's long terminal illness. In addition, he likely would have met the psychiatric criteria for post-traumatic stress disorder in the period following the death of his father during the Lightning Way ceremony years before. Incidentally, he reportedly had a history of cruelty to animals and a lot of "running around" behavior with alcohol use and his multiple "wives," though in the absence of a criminal history this does not add up to an antisocial personality.

Following the ceremony, which took place over the course of a weekend and included two of his sisters as copatients, Jesse slept the night in the hogan where it took place, beginning a period of four days in which a patient is supposed to remain still and reverent. He reported feeling that the ceremony had gone well. When asked what had been the most important part, he said, "the whole thing." He said he was not feeling or thinking about much during the ceremony, just focusing on the proceedings. He did, however, mention being nervous throughout: "I felt like I was just a bundle of nerves," he said. "Maybe that was the workings of the tobacco and the mixing of the herbs working on me together," but mostly, as they worked, the tobacco and the herbs combined to make "my whole being [feel] fine." Jesse also said he had a hard time following and repeating the chanter's prayers, a fundamental aspect of the traditional patient's participation. He indicated that he thought the ceremony would help him, but he also qualified this by saying it was best not to be too confident. He said that having faith in healing was very important: "They say you have to have complete faith, that is the only way you get healed, that's what they say. The Holy People [i.e., the traditional Navajo deities, or *yei*] are like that, you have to believe in them for them to help you. The same way with God." His attitude might be called one of faithful but cautious optimism. "You have to take caution here," he said. "You can't shout and say, I'm all well, and it's pretty good. You might be lying. Then you wonder if they were truthful. It's up to the Holy People." Like most traditional people, he felt that a cure does not come immediately but rather will come with time:

> When you suffer from such an event, and you come down life's road, and you suffer all kinds of things from it. This suffering, in itself, is a teaching tool. . . . And now, finally, I had this Lightning Way ceremony performed, and now, it seems like someone has said, "Wait, wait." That's how it seems to me. In a few days, after four days, I'm sure everything will be fine. It is at that point that you become a real believer. Right now you do believe too, and it has helped you too.

Once that healing occurs, one's belief is strengthened, and out of suffering comes understanding.

Following the Lightning Way ceremony, Jesse reported that he was no longer feeling hot all the time and breaking out into a sweat spontaneously. By two weeks after the ceremony, he told us that his vision had gotten better, and the difficulties he had been having while walking seemed to have disappeared, though he also mentioned the persistence of pain ("it feels like it has pins and needles") in his feet, especially in his heels. He said that working around his farm, which had been very difficult for him before the ceremony, had gotten easier for him. "It seems to be going in the healing direction for me, yes," he told us. At a follow-up interview three months later, however, things were much different, and he had had more difficulties. He indicated that his recent ceremony was somewhat invalidated by two occurrences. First, he had seen and killed a snake within a few days of the ceremony, significant both in ritual terms and with respect to his apparent ambivalence regarding such violations of convention. Second, he had a personal tragedy when a nephew who had passed out drunk on train tracks was run over by a train. This death figured importantly in Jesse's healing process, because the chanter had warned him and his family against having anything to do with the dead. Unfortunately, after the accident, the nephew's body was returned and his sisters hugged it in grief. Jesse believed that this in itself undid the effects of the ceremony, not just for his sisters, but for him as well. He specifically mentioned that his own pain had returned after this incident.

As a result of this incident, the Lightning Way chanter told Jesse that he should get rediagnosed and have another ceremony. Jesse said he was planning on having this chanter complete another full ceremony for him, "when I am financially able to." In addition, he said that he still needed a full Evil Way ceremony following the death of his second wife:

> My late wife used to live here and be present here. Her presence is all over the place, her hand body oils are still on everything. She still has some of her personal possessions around in the house, there is one over there. Maybe that is what is affecting the house. Because of that, I won't move back in until the hogan has been properly cleaned. Then I will live in here again. Now, I'm being told to get well first, and sleep over at the other house for the time being. That is what my older sister tells me to do. She will clean this hogan out first, before I will move back in here.

In conjunction with this concern, Jesse was worried that some of her health difficulties may have been related to, or caused by, his own past disrespect for the values, attitudes, and rules of the Holy People. Finally, he was concerned that he had seen and killed a snake immediately following his recent ceremony. He thought the appearance of the snake meant that someone was trying to witch him or, as he put it, that someone was "still" trying to witch him, intimating as well that witchcraft likely played a role in the death of his latest wife.

Let us formulate the therapeutic process experienced by Jesse with respect to the rhetorical model outlined above. Jesse had a positive disposition toward healing, but his faith and optimism were tempered by his idea that too strong an expectation to be healed could be a setup for failure and might incur disfavor with the Holy People. In addition, he expressed a theme of having many ceremonies but not being fully integrated by them, as well as a theme of ambivalence toward ritual conventions, the violation of which could undermine ceremonial efficacy.

In a number of instances in which ceremonies had not cured or even helped him, he was critical of the healers — either he regarded the traditional diagnosticians as frauds or felt that the chanters omitted certain key features of the rite and their omission caused the cure to fail. The failure of these ceremonies quite likely caused him to have some caution about the imminence of a cure. Like many traditional people, Jesse felt that a cure could be a long time in coming, implicitly suggesting that the therapeutic process is lifelong. From his comments, it does not appear that Jesse expects his ceremonies to end the troubles that stem from an event that happened over forty years ago. The effects of the lightning strike implicated his entire family and will continue to affect them throughout their lives. Realistically, he is hoping for relief from his symptoms. He feels that even if his condition improves in the short run, he will need to have additional ceremonies. Another salient fact with regard to Jesse's disposition toward healing is an apparent willingness to disregard ritual proscriptions even as he maintains a belief in them. This may reflect an attitude that when one does something wrong, punishment may or may not result, an attitude that often leads people not to have ceremonies until something goes wrong. Finally, Jesse's disposition included the possibility of a partial cure. He had a plethora of symptoms, some that he reported improved and others that remained the same. Nevertheless, by the time of our follow-up interview, other events had occurred that he saw as undermining his ceremony, events that did not concern him directly but his sisters, who had been copatients in the ceremony. In his opinion, their contact with the dead was enough to undo his ceremony.

Our interviews suggest that Jesse has a vivid sense of the sacred and a life suffused with the sacred dimensions of traditional Navajo religion — the repercussions of broken ritual proscriptions, ceremonials, prayer, witchcraft, "skinwalkers," etc. His experience of the sacred in the ceremony itself also seems to have been strong. He said on several occasions that the ritual use of herbs and tobacco altered his mind and body in a positive way. His expressed fear that his inability to repeat the prayer properly might cause problems for him also suggests his belief that the Holy People are tangible and, because this ceremony was properly performed with all the necessary elements, were present and would hear his prayers. A final episode that suggests a high degree of sacred experience in Jesse's case is his contact with a snake in the aftermath of the ceremony. He agreed that this was probably a bad sign and, cognizant of his own past with both lightning and snakes, must have seen it as meaningful. Nevertheless, it was not the snake but his sisters' contact with the dead to which he attributed the undoing of his ceremony. Moreover, he did not associate the snake with his own behavior but read it as a witchcraft attempt by others.

With respect to the elaborations of alternatives, Jesse sees not a series of behavioral or emotional possibilities before him but a variety of ceremonial possibilities, as well as a variety of possible outcomes ranging from success, to partial success, to failure. In addition to the Lightning Way ceremony, he felt he still needed an Evil Way because of the death of his wife and an Enemy Way to remove the white woman's remains from the car he cleaned out. He seemed quite sure that he had needed all the components that had been included in the Lightning Way, such as the offering and the rinsing in addition to the sand-painting, since a diagnostician had told him that the reason past ceremonies failed was that some of these had been omitted. Jesse's story and the particular sense it gives to the notion of an elaboration of alternatives highlights a powerful theme in traditional Navajo therapeutic process, namely, contamination via contact — with lightning, with a variety of animals, with the dead, with his dying second wife, sexually with his first wife, with the dead "enemy," or with a witch or "skinwalker."

Actualization of change is both tentative and incremental in Jesse's case. Despite his feeling that the ceremony went very well, he was initially reluctant to regard the healing as a success, because such optimism could cause problems. Nevertheless, his interviews are punctuated with positive statements about its effects. These range from alleviation of pain and improvement of physical symptoms to an improvement in his outlook and the ability to get up earlier and get his farm work done. Again, there are other symptoms, specifically some pain in his legs and feet, which he did not feel had disappeared and had improved marginally at best. Three months later, things had changed somewhat because of the violent death of a nephew and his copatients' subsequent contact with the corpse. It is difficult to regard this as an unrelated event, however, since it is of a kind that has a direct bearing on the therapeutic process, insofar as that process merges with a person's overall life trajectory.

Conclusion

In this chapter, I have offered two accounts of the experiential specificity of the therapeutic process in ritual healing. In these accounts, we are already a long way from the phenomenological muteness in some abstract accounts of healing. Likewise, we are far from the black box of mechanisms such as suggestion, catharsis, or trance, often put forward to account for the efficacy of spiritual healing. Both approaches characterize the classic case described by Claude Lévi-Strauss of the Cuna Indian ritual, in which he hypothesized that the distress of giving birth was ameliorated by the combination of abstract homology between the structure of the shaman's chant and the structure of the physiological process of labor, and the ritual's triggering of an abreaction and catharsis for the patient.[4] Our method of eliciting experiential commentary allows us to achieve a greater degree of specificity than is typically available in such accounts. It allows us to monitor incremental change in self and suffering by describing the embodied-self process of healing with respect to the therapeutic functions of disposition, experience of the sacred, elaboration of alternatives, and actualization of change. Following each patient over time also allows us to understand how therapeutic process transcends the boundaries of particular sessions and permeates the pursuit of everyday life concerns.

Finally, it invites us to compare, on both existential and spiritual grounds, the dimensions of compatibility and incommensurability in which humanity encounters suffering and strives for its amelioration. In fact, the symptoms of these two patients in terms of somatic pathology and psychopathology are quite divergent, as are the cosmological and theological underpinnings of the healing systems in which they engage. It is in the moral domain where we find a common ground or, in Arthur Kleinman's phrase, all that really matters, in experiential and interpersonal terms.[5] This is the locus of phenomenological and human convergence in these otherwise dissimilar accounts.

The competing demands for high levels of personal achievement and emotionally engaged marital intimacy is precisely a moral dilemma for the man with the German general within. It is safe to say that within contemporary North American culture, the stereotypic image of the German general refers explicitly to a Nazi general. The patient referred to the inner controller subpersonality as a "Gestapo type" — adding the moral connotation of cruelty to that of excessive discipline. The effects of this cruelty were felt not so much by the patient himself — who, after all, found a kind of satisfaction in the compulsion to achieve — but in his marital relationship and the emotional deprivation of his wife. In all this, it is critical to recognize that the moral element is embedded not in a discourse of sin and culpability but in the idiom of suffering, affliction, and healing as is characteristic of the ethos of Charismatic Christianity. The imaginal performance itself consisted essentially of a moral *entente* between the subpersonality and the patient, mediated by the divine figure of Jesus and taking place in a peaceful garden.

---

4. See Claude Lévi-Strauss, *Structural Anthropology* (New York: Basic, 1966), esp. 181–201.

5. See Arthur Kleinman, *What Really Matters: Living a Moral Life amidst Uncertainty and Danger* (Oxford: Oxford University Press, 2007).

The man struck by lightning was no less faced with a moral dilemma. If on first thought his affliction appears to stem from violation of an abstract and impersonal cosmological ritual proscription associated with the power of lightning, on second thought what is clearly at issue is moral in two explicit senses. Most immediately, his wife violated this ritual proscription when she failed to observe what Navajos refer to as the period of reverence following a ceremony, and she carelessly and selfishly exposed herself to a force that, out of its proper ceremonial place, was a source of contamination and danger. In addition, this action was not only heedless of the potentially dangerous spiritual power of a natural force, but a natural force understood to be analogous to that of the Holy People or deities. The problem is not so much that the deity responds by taking offense and out of revenge causes affliction — as might be the case with Olympian deities or Yoruba Orixas — but that the action disrupts the natural order of the world that is itself a sentient world continuous with that of human sensibility. Ambivalence toward ritual proscriptions is in this sense a trope for ambivalence toward moral conventions, and an apparently impersonal stricture has immediate implications in the interpersonal realm. Thus killing a snake is not simply a violation of the snake as a holy being but is also complicated by the understanding of the snake as an emissary of witchery by hostile others. Intimate contact with the dead is not simply tempting supernatural harassment by ghosts but also violates conventions for the ethically appropriate management of grief due to bereavement.

Can we address the question whether these healing systems and these particular cases of healing are genuine and authentic? Perhaps this question is poorly phrased since, in a way, it evokes a notion that is almost commercial — is this bag a genuine Versace, is this painting an authentic van Gogh, is this ceremony a genuine act of healing? The question of authenticity in healing is better put in terms of whether the system has the symbolic and pragmatic capacity to address human suffering and, on the level of an individual case, whether the participants are sincere in their engagement with the attempt to alleviate suffering. In this respect, the question of efficacy is not one of active ingredients versus placebos, of faith versus doubt, or of magic versus science, but one of theodicy and morality. In the Christian system, God allows suffering as a consequence of primordial disloyalty on the part of human beings, but those forms of Christianity that entertain the possibility of ritual healing suggest that God allows suffering only to a certain point. God decides whether to heal. In the Navajo system, the world originally included a large number of monsters that afflicted humans, such that suffering is a part of being. Fortunately, most were eliminated by the mythical hero twins Monster Slayer and Born for Water, but several managed to survive — including, Disease, Death, Hunger, and Violence. Things would have been worse without these heroes. In the moral domain, Christians are obligated to be moral out of devotion to God, in imitation of God, or at least to avoid the omnipotent deity's wrath. In the Navajo Way, the Holy People can be compelled to act by appropriate ceremonial means, and, in concordance with what John Ladd identified as "atomic egoism," moral acts will have favorable consequences on the actor, and immoral acts unfavorable consequences.[6]

Is there a continuity between anthropological and theological assessments of healing? If not, what is the nature of the disjunction, and if so, where does one begin and the other leave off? Perhaps the most obvious difference is that theology has less of a tendency toward comparativism, while anthropology is inveterately comparative. To invoke comparativism is not the same as invoking relativism, for suffering and evil are bedrock universals of the human condition. The comparative approach, however, must begin with an acknowledgment that the encounter with suffering and healing has permutations depending on whether a deity is monotheistic, omnipotent, and universal, or whether the spiritual world is defined by a personified pantheism in which every discrete phenomenon has its own identity and integrity within the order of things and beings.

One way to address this question is to consider the difference between the notions of miracle and meaning. In less-than-subtle terms, theology might look for a miracle, while anthropology might deny the miraculous in favor of a naturalistic notion of spontaneous remission. Theology might say that meaning is to be found in the mercy of God, while anthropology might say that meaning is to be found in the transformative power of the human imagination. Neither of these attributions is quite fair to the discipline in question. It is likely that a mature theology would not require a dramatic miracle as necessary in the assessment of healing, on the grounds that a very small change can be as profound and compelling as a big one and that a transformation of meaning can be just as miraculous as the banishment of symptoms. It is likely that a mature anthropology could understand the spiritual value drawn from a spontaneous remission by the participants in ritual healing and that the human imagination is a divine function by any definition of the term.

Already more than four decades ago, Erika Bourguignon observed that the efficacy of religious healing is to be found most often not in the removal of a disease and its symptoms but in transforming the meaning of an illness.[7] This is

---

6. John Ladd, *The Structure of a Moral Code: A Philosophical Analysis of Ethical Discourse Applied to the Ethics of the Navaho Indians* (Cambridge, MA: Harvard University Press, 1957).

7. Erika Bourguignon, "The Effectiveness of Religious Healing Movements," *Transcultural Psychiatric Research Review* 12 (1976): 5–21.

no retreat into ambiguity but a penetrating insight into the human condition. Meaning is not the exclusive domain of anthropology, theology, or any other discipline but pertains equally to all scholarship that inquires into the existential, moral, and spiritual grounds of human life. This is why the comparative study of healing can teach us so much, for it is an exquisite display of meaning-making that has the potential to transform self and social relations in the most incremental or the most profound ways.[8]

8. Thanks to Sarah Coakley for her editorial advice, to Arthur Kleinman for encouraging me to draw out the moral dimensions of the comparison, and to Janis Jenkins for her critical insight and emotional sustenance throughout every phase of this work.

IO

Healing in Pastoral Care

John Swinton

Hard on the heels of an anthropological account of the meaning systems of healing, we come, finally, to an explicitly *theological* reflection on how healing operates within the parallel systems of Christian pastoral care.

And so here we ask once more: What does it *mean* to be healed? As one who reflects on the wide panoply of understandings of the term *healing*, it soon becomes clear that answering such an apparently simple question is not straightforward. Does healing mean cure? Is it physical, psychological, or spiritual? Does it mean learning to look at your problem or illness differently? Is it something that belongs firmly within the domain of medicine? Or is it essentially a supernatural event that is a divine reward for achieving adequate levels of faithfulness? Even if one modifies the term *healing* with *Christian*, the polyvalence of meaning does not necessarily decrease. And yet, despite the confusion, the question of what it means to be healed remains of great significance to the pastoral ministry of the church. Among the world's religions, Christianity differs in its supreme emphasis on healing. Jesus's healing miracles were central to his identity and ministry (see chapter 1) and vital for the communication of his revelation of the God of compassion and grace who brings unmerited healing to a broken world. Healing matters for Christians. And yet not all are healed, at least not if we define healing in terms of cure. Some are healed, and some are not. Why is this so? If healing is so central to Christianity, then why is the practice of healing so apparently inconsistent and unpredictable? What are we doing, and what should we expect when we engage in Christian healing practices?

In this chapter, I want to offer a perspective on Christian spiritual healing that will begin to tease out possible answers to questions such as these and offer an understanding of spiritual healing that presents interesting possibilities for the pastoral ministry and the churches' ministry of healing.

What Does Christian Healing Mean?

For the purposes of this section of the chapter, I use the term *spiritual healing* to refer to healing that occurs via a seemingly direct intervention from God. I begin with these presuppositions — born out of my own experiences and those of people close to me — that God does indeed heal today (healing here understood in terms of cure) and that supernatural intervention is possible, although it is not predictable or controllable. I do not intend to work out the mechanics of Christian supernatural healing. I am content to leave the how and the why to God. My primary interest in the first section of this chapter, however, is in the *meaning* of spiritual healing. The question that I want to begin with is this: In the strange marketplace of healing alternatives, precisely what does Christian healing mean? It is important to note that I am asking not what Christian healing *is*. My interest is in the question of what Christian healing *means*. The difference is important. The former question seeks explanation; the latter seeks understanding. My approach is therefore hermeneutical in its focus and intention.

Hermeneutics as a Tool of Exploration

In order to begin to answer this question, we need some tools and perspectives that will allow us to access the vital meaning dimensions of Christian healing, dimensions that are often overlooked when we insist on focusing only on end points that demand cure as the primary source of validation for the churches' healing practices. Unless we understand the nature of and reason for the journey, the destination will be at best confusing and at worst damaging. Indeed, as we shall see, the hermeneutical journey that *is* healing may actually be more important than outcomes that are defined by desires that are limited to what we might hope cure to look like.

Hermeneutics is a generic term for various theories of interpretation. Richard Palmer defines hermeneutics as the process wherein "something foreign, strange, or separated in time, space, or experience is revealed so as to seem familiar and comprehensible. . . . Language is the medium par excellence in this process."[1] A hermeneutical perspective assumes that there is no access to reality that is not interpreted. Human beings are constantly creating and recreating the world through the process of interpretation. A hermeneutical perspective is, therefore, always suspicious of truth claims that are proposed as timeless, universal givens. While ultimate truths may well exist, they are always processed via a complex matrix of hermeneutical contexts and processes. As Al Dowie puts it, hermeneutics "modifies epistemology towards the provisionality of knowledge across a range of Knowing."[2] Within this perspective, claims about reality are understood as the product of a process of epistemological negotiation that goes on within particular individuals, communities, cultures, and subcultures across the breadth of human experience.

The history of hermeneutics is complex and diverse, as are the multitude of theoretical perspectives that have emerged as people seek to interpret the world. For current purposes, my focus here will be on one particular theory of hermeneutics that is helpful in throwing light on the meaning of Christian healing: the hermeneutical theory of the German philosopher, Hans-Georg Gadamer. For Gadamer, hermeneutics is more than simply something that human beings do; it is something that human beings *are*. As he puts it, understanding is "not just one of the various possible behaviors of the subject, but the mode of being."[3] Hermeneutics, then, is more than epistemology; it is ontological in nature. Despite the fact that it is often used in this way, Gadamer's project was not to develop a methodology for the human sciences.[4] Rather his intention was to clarify the conditions in which understanding can take place.[5] His intention was to expose what is wrong with the type of thinking that moves between the poles of objectivity and relativism and to open up a new way of thinking about understanding.[6]

"Prejudice"

Gadamer assumes that when we confront a text, we do so with a particular preunderstanding that emerges from and is rooted in some form of common culture and history that is embedded in language. We can make sense of action

1. Richard Palmer, *Hermeneutics* (Evanston, IL: Northwestern University Press, 1969), 13.
2. Al Dowie, *Interpreting Culture in a Scottish Congregation* (New York: Peter Lang, 2002), 12.
3. Hans-Georg Gadamer, *Truth and Method* (London: Sheed and Ward, 1975), xviii.
4. Gadamer, *Truth and Method*, xiii.
5. Gadamer, *Truth and Method*, 265.
6. R. J. Bernstein, *Beyond Objectivism and Relativism* (Philadelphia: University of Pennsylvania Press, 1983), 34-38.

only in terms of the values, virtues, and story of the good life that prevail within our cultural world. He refers to these preunderstandings as *prejudices*.[7] His use of the term *prejudice* should not be perceived as negative. Quite the opposite, our prejudices are the key to the way that we come to understand the world. Hekman describes Gadamer's idea of prejudice as a "forestructure or a condition of knowledge in that it determines what we may find intelligible in any given situation. [Gadamer] replaces the opposition between truth and prejudice with the assertion that prejudice — our situatedness in history and time — is the precondition of truth, not an obstacle to it."[8] Our prejudices are therefore very important for the process of interpretation and understanding. Indeed, we can access the world only through our prejudices. Gadamer puts it thus:

> a hermeneutically trained mind must be, from the start, sensitive to the text's quality of newness. But this kind of sensitivity involves neither "neutrality" in the matter of the object nor the extinction of one's self, but the conscious assimilation of one's own foremeaning and prejudices. The important thing is to be aware of one's own bias, so that the text may present itself in all its newness and thus be able to assert its own truth against one's own foremeanings. (238)

Understanding thus takes place in the dialogical interplay between the text we seek to understand and our own prejudices. If we fail to recognize the influence of either of these aspects, we risk misunderstanding the meaning of the text. "[It] is the tyranny of hidden prejudices that makes us deaf to the language that speaks to us" (239). In order to understand and assimilate new experiences, it is necessary to draw on this preunderstanding. Therefore, in contrast to the assumptions of objectivism, prejudice — our situatedness in history and time — is the precondition of truth rather than an obstacle to it. Thus, the basic structure of a person or a community's effective history constrains and to an extent defines the range of possible interpretations, excluding some possibilities and calling forth others.[9] It is, therefore, necessary for persons to be aware of their own historical situatedness and the ways that this influences their interpretations of

7. Gadamer, *Truth and Method*, 238. Hereafter, page references to this book will be given in parentheses in the text.

8. S. Hekman, *Hermeneutics and the Sociology of Knowledge* (Cambridge: Polity, 1986), 117.

9. In this sense, hermeneutics can be understood as tradition-informed inquiry, insofar as questions that are being investigated are always viewed not only in their cultural-historical context but also from the context or tradition of the interpreter. We cannot step outside culture and history. Actions make sense only as they interact with our presumptions about what is valuable and virtuous.

those texts, objects, people, and events they seek to understand.[10] The "historically effective consciousness" is one that is truly open to experience and that
is aware of the influence of a person's and a culture's preunderstandings of the
ways they see the world (204ff.).

The Fusion of Horizons

A second Gadamerian concept that is of importance for the current investigation is the idea of the fusion of horizons. This links closely with the idea of
prejudice and functions in like manner to a hermeneutical circle. The prejudices and foremeanings that form the mind and cultural worldview of the interpreter — those concepts and understandings that make understanding possible — are deeply bound to the *horizon* of the interpreter. "Understanding is not
to be thought of so much as an action of one's subjectivity, but as the placing of
oneself within a process of tradition, in which past and present are constantly
fused" (258).

Gadamer describes this process of "placing oneself within a process of tradition" as the fusion of horizons: "The wide superior vision that the person
who is seeking to understand must have; to acquire a horizon means that one
learns to look beyond what is close at hand — not in order to look away from
it, but to see it better within a larger whole and in truer proportion" (275). The
horizon of the interpreter includes her entire forestructure with all its inherent
prejudices, that is, what we find intelligible given our specific cultural perspectives and our place in history. Put slightly differently, the horizon includes
everything that can be seen from a particular vantage point within history
and tradition. It contains nothing beyond that. Gadamer's point is not that,
in order to understand, we somehow need to reach out and locate ourselves
within a different horizon or another historical situation or tradition. Such a
task is clearly impossible (269–73). We cannot leave our own horizon. But we
can merge our horizons with the horizons of others. Indeed, any developing
tradition requires or, better, depends on an ongoing process of assimilating
new interpretations and perspectives (358). Understanding occurs when the
horizon of the interpreter intersects or fuses with the horizon of the object of
inquiry. Within this dialogical process, there is a realization that the range of
interpretations of a particular text or situation is broad and diverse. Understanding is never actually complete.

---

10. For a further development of this point, see my *Spirituality and Mental Health Care:
Rediscovering a 'Forgotten' Dimension* (London: Jessica Kingsley, 2001), ch. 4.

A Full or a Partial Hermeneutic?

Gadamer's hermeneutical perspective will enable us to begin to move toward an answer to our key question: What does Christian healing *mean*? However, we cannot take Gadamer's hermeneutics on board uncritically. His hermeneutic is what might be described as a *full* hermeneutic. It assumes that all human understanding is bound to and mediated by cultural and historical contexts, what he describes as *effective history* (personal experience and cultural traditions). For Gadamer, there can be no single meaning and no core of truth that can be accessed in an uninterpreted form. Such a full hermeneutic poses problems for those who adhere to a tradition such as Christianity that makes concrete truth claims. Christianity assumes that God (Truth) is in fact accessible in a form that, while clearly influenced by human interpretation, in a very real sense transcends its vicissitudes. Christians believe not only that truth is real and objectively verifiable — paradigmatically in the life, death, and resurrection of Jesus — but also that it is available to human beings via divine revelation. Certainly that accessibility is clouded and affected by culture, tradition, history, and sin, but accessing aspects of the truth of God remains a firm possibility. I would therefore, on such theological grounds, be wary of accepting the full hermeneutic that Gadamer espouses.

That being so, I would wish to hold on to the essence of Gadamer's position but step back from the fullness of his hermeneutical position to one of *critical realism*.[11] Critical realism takes seriously the insights offered by Gadamer's full hermeneutical perspective but, while recognizing the provisional nature of human perceptions of reality, does not regard truth as totally inaccessible. Prejudice and history are acknowledged as vital to the process of interpretation, but the assumption remains that truth is available, albeit in a form that emerges through and always remains embedded in human constructions. The perspective that underpins this chapter accepts the notion that the idea of value-free, objective truth is problematic and probably unsustainable. Nevertheless, it continues to acknowledge that reality in general, and divine reality in particular, can be known a little better through our constructions, even if, at the same time, we must acknowledge that some of our constructions remain provisional and open to challenge. In other words, there may be better or worse descriptions of the reality, but there is reality that can be grasped. The aim of this critical-realist hermeneutic is not objectivity and absolute certainty but forms of *understanding* that enable us to see the world a little more clearly. With these hermeneutical insights in mind, we can now proceed with our reflections on the meaning of Christian healing.

11. R. Bhaskar, *A Realist Theory of Science*, 2nd ed. (London: Verso, 1997).

The Power of Prejudice: Rethinking Health and Healing

As we have seen, Gadamer is clear that it is through our prejudices that we are enabled to make sense of our world. Of course, many of our prejudices are not encountered at a conscious level. They are deeply engrained in our worldview, often in ways that we are barely conscious of until they are brought to our attention. Our worldviews make up our perspective on and understanding of the world. They contain and define the structures of normality and general assumptions about the nature of reality for individuals and cultures. They provide the plausibility structures within which personal and cultural definitions of reality are worked out and sustained.[12] Importantly, worldviews shape what we see in the world and influence the ways we act on the world. In other words, the forms of action that we take in response to our experiences in the world are determined by the way we interpret and understand the world to be. Worldviews are not real in a strictly ontological sense. Worldviews are always temporary and are constantly changing. We no longer believe that the earth is flat or that the sun revolves around the earth. But we did at a particular moment in history; at one time, it was considered to be a scientific fact. Presumably much of the knowledge we currently have will also be shown to be false at some point in the future. Worldviews are thus temporary and transient. Worldviews *are* nevertheless real for those who accept them.

At any given point, particular dominant ideas shape worldviews and the thinking and understandings of those who accept them as reality. For example, Cartesian philosophy has profoundly impacted Western thinking and understandings about the essence of humanness; science and the scientific method have deeply influenced the ways we access and validate truth and reality; religion has and continues to be a powerful force in shaping our understanding of the nature and possibility of transcendence. In our present time, biomedicine has become a powerful shaper of our worldview, particularly with regard to the ways we understand health, disease, and healing, so much so that it is almost impossible for us to think about health and illness without first thinking about medicine. There may well be a wide range of healing alternatives, but biomedicine remains culturally prized above most others.

The roots of biomedicine lie in the emergence of science and reason during the Enlightenment. Its healing techniques, assumptions, and practices have a charac-

---

12. See, for example, Peter Berger, *The Sacred Canopy* (New York: Doubleday, 1967), and Peter Berger, B. Berger, and H. Kellner, *The Homeless Mind: Modernization and Consciousness* (New York: Penguin, 1974).

teristic shape that, Colin Samson argues, has emerged as a result of the scientism and empiricism of the Enlightenment: "Enlightenment medicine reflected a confidence in scientific methods of observation and experimentation to *control* nature and *intervene* to correct ailments that seemed to cut short life.... The approach to sickness advocated by the medical profession has now become almost a monopoly by virtue of its legitimisation by the state in all Western countries as well as other societies."[13] Within this approach to healing, health is understood primarily in biological terms and illness perceived as something that requires taming through medical technological intervention. Wigg refers to this approach to healing as "techno-medicine," an approach to medicine within which "the questions related to the moral and spiritual side of the individual are considered merely as frills of culture and have no place in an economically driven scientific regime."[14] Interestingly, Wigg argues that the dominance of "techno-medicine" has resulted in a redefinition of the issues that once preoccupied philosophers:

What is human nature?
How is happiness achieved?
What is a good life?

These questions have been restated as:

What is normal?
How can it be measured?
What conclusions are generalizable?

Within this cultural milieu, the question of what healing *means* makes little sense.

The biomedical model that emerged from the development of biomedicine and that has come to dominate our understandings of health, illness, and healing has three underlying assumptions and principles. First, it assumes the centrality of *objectivism*. Objectivism presupposes that for knowledge to be accurate, it must be achieved through an instantiated and impersonal assessment of information that is received via the senses. Second, *determinism* assumes that causality must be presupposed to be mechanical and linear. Third, the idea of *positivism* assumes that genuine knowledge can be acquired only through applying the scientific method to experiences through the process of observation

---

13. Colin Samson, *Health Studies: A Critical and Cross-Cultural Reader* (London: Blackwell, 1999), 3.

14. N. N. Wigg, "Plenary Lecture Delivered at the Mary Hemingway Rees Memorial Lecture" (World Federation of Mental Health, Trinity College, Dublin, August 1995), 298.

via the senses. Forms of metaphysical speculation are rejected by positivism as they are not verifiable through the scientific method.

Within this epistemological framework, physical and psychological disorders are assumed to have a fixed form. Disease is assumed to have the following:

1. a *specific etiology* — that is, disease is located within particular and identifiable pathological structures within discrete human bodies;
2. a *predictable course*; and
3. *describable signs and symptoms*, which is to say, a predictable outcome modifiable by certain technical maneuvers.

Here disease is identified as a discrete "bad spot" within an individual that needs to be excised or at least controlled by medical technology. Health is defined in terms of the absence of pathology, and healing is defined primarily in terms of a movement toward cure. What is interesting about the approach of the medical model is that, in principle at least, there is no need for the presence of a person. The idea of individuals as meaningful beings with goals, dreams, expectations, and hopes is substituted for an understanding of persons as machines or at least as machine-like. Within this understanding, good healers are perceived as effective mechanics able to utilize scientific technology to bring the body back to a state of health and well-being.

The biomedical approach to health and illness is so basic to our prejudices as we approach the issues surrounding Christian healing that it is difficult for us to separate our own horizons from the very different horizon that Scripture gives us in its healing narratives. Take for example Jesus's healing of the leper, as it is recounted in Mark's Gospel:

> A leper came to him begging him, and kneeling he said to him, "If you choose, you can make me clean." Moved with pity, Jesus stretched out his hand and touched him, and said to him, "I do choose. Be made clean!" Immediately the leprosy left him, and he was made clean. After sternly warning him he sent him away at once, saying to him, "See that you say nothing to anyone; but go, show yourself to the priest, and offer for your cleansing what Moses commanded, as a testimony to them." But he went out and began to proclaim it freely, and to spread the word, so that Jesus could no longer go into a town openly, but stayed out in the country; and people came to him from every quarter. (Mark 1:40–45)

As we read this story, we inevitably find ourselves reflecting on the *disease* of leprosy (the bad spot) and the method of excising the disease that Jesus used to *cure*

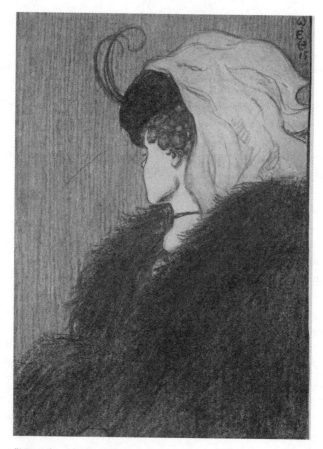

*"My wife and my mother-in-law. They are both in this picture —
find them" by W. E. Hill.*

the man with leprosy (the spiritual healing). We may pay lip service to the other
social and theological dimensions within the story, but within the actual practice
of healing as it is now taught and carried out within the contemporary church, it is
often the physical outcome (the cure) that people tend to focus on. Our biomedical prejudice inevitably impinges upon our efforts to understand precisely what Jesus was doing and how we can most effectively bring our horizons of understanding into successful fusion with an action that took place within Mediterranean
culture around two thousand years ago; again, this is a very different horizon.

However, if we are not aware of the boundaries and limitations of our own
horizon and if our horizon is impervious to challenge or change, we risk missing

out on the crucial inner theological *meaning* (as opposed to the outcome) of such instances of spiritual healing. Such misinterpretation can lead to pastoral practices and approaches that can be deeply damaging. The optical illusion on page 214 will help illustrate the point.

The problem here is that *people in general tend to see what* they *expect to see* (i.e., what their prejudices have led them to presume about a particular event, experience, or situation). You will probably be familiar with the optical illusion above. It illustrates well the significance of Gadamer's ideas about prejudice and effective history. Where you have been (your history) shapes what you *expect* to see. If you have a historical context that includes young women as a prominent theme, you will see the young woman. If your historical context has attuned you toward older women, then that is what you will see. Eventually you will become aware of both horizons, and also the reality that you need to understand the whole of the picture in order to understand the parts. However, most people do not see the whole until the second one is pointed out to them. I want to suggest that a similar process is at work in the ways we understand health and healing. Because biomedicine is such a powerful aspect of our worldview (such a major influence on our horizon), at least in the West, it is very difficult for us to see disease and healing in any other way until an alternative is pointed out. When this new horizon is pointed out to us, we cannot but begin to see things differently and, in seeing differently, begin to act differently.

Reframing Spiritual Healing

Good and Good make an important observation: "All illness realities [are] fundamentally semantic. . . . Whatever the biological correlates or grounds of a disease, sickness becomes a human experience and an object of therapeutic attention as it is made meaningful. . . . *All* illness realities are meaningfully constituted."[15] All disease processes are open to a multitude of different interpretations and explanations. The way that a disease is interpreted will determine the method of healing that is employed and legitimized within particular contexts and cultures. Within Western cultures, we have *chosen* (it is important to note that this is a cultural *choice* and not an inevitability) to interpret disease primarily in terms of the biomedical model's emphasis on observable objective

---

15. B. Good and M. Good, "The Meaning of Symptoms: A Cultural Hermeneutic Model for Clinical Practice," in *The Relevance of Social Science for Medicine*, ed. L. Eisenberg and A. Kleinman (Norwell, MA: Kluwer, 1988), 167.

pathology. This is not, however, the only way we can understand disease and healing. Biomedical eyes are automatically drawn to the story of the healing of the leper as a miraculous physical healing of an individual with an identifiable pathology (such a description is not of course inaccurate, just inadequate).[16] However, if we allow ourselves to become aware of our prejudices and the limitations of our horizon and begin to allow that horizon to merge with the horizon of the culture within which this healing took place, things begin to look a little different.

John Pilch notes that the main problem with leprosy within first-century Mediterranean culture was not the specific pathology of the condition or even the fear of contagion. In all the stories that mention the healing of leprosy, lepers seem to have free access to Jesus. Contagion was clearly not the major issue. Rather, the real issue was *pollution and a threat to holiness*.[17] To have leprosy was to be perceived as religiously impure and, as such, to be excluded from the forms of worship and ritual cleansing that enabled one to relate directly to God and to participate within the worshiping community. Without such a relationship, people remained in their sinful condition with no possibility of redemption. People with this condition were considered nonpersons in the eyes of society and culture and, so it was assumed, also in the eyes of God. Within a society where one's personhood — as constituted by its individual, social, and spiritual dimensions — depended on being affirmed by and incorporated within the community and ultimately reconciled with God, exclusion from that community would have been as painful as the sores of the medical condition, if not more so.[18] In other words, the problem with leprosy was a *theological* one, which included, but was not defined by, its medical aspects.

Understood from this perspective, Jesus's healing actions were not primarily medical or therapeutic, at least not in the contemporary sense in which these terms are used. Rather, they were acts of theological and social transformation designed to cleanse and revalidate the individual and, in so doing, open up previously closed access to God and to the Jewish and nascent Christian communities. It is not insignificant that in the gospel reports on the healing of leprosy, Jesus *touches* the sick person. At one level, the touch mediated God's healing

16. See, for example, John Wilkinson, *The Bible and Healing: A Medical and Theological Commentary* (Grand Rapids: Eerdmans, 2000).

17. John Pilch, *Healing in the New Testament: Insights from Medical Anthropology* (Minneapolis: Fortress, 2002), 52.

18. For an important reflection on the difference between disease, pain, and suffering, see Eric Cassel's *The Nature of Suffering and the Goals of Medicine* (New York: Oxford University Press, 1991).

power. But perhaps, at least in the healing of leprosy, Jesus's touch physically symbolizes an acceptance back into community. If we are right in thinking that the problem with leprosy was the socially constructed experience of pollution rather than contagion, then the problem is found to lie within the *community* rather than within the boundaries of the man's body. The presence of a leprous person in the community was perceived as somehow polluting the community. Jesus's touching the leper demonstrates in a concrete way that the individual is a full member of the community *as Jesus understands it*. Jesus, who is God, not only facilitates the reincorporation of the individual back into the community; he also challenges the community to rethink what it means to be the community of a God who touches lepers. In a profound and theologically significant way, the community refuses to touch that which God, in Jesus, embraces — thus, ironically, excluding itself from God's presence. In touching this person, Jesus challenges the community to recognize who God is and, in so doing, to mirror God's healing actions revealed in Jesus. By doing so, the community is given the opportunity to become a place of faithfulness where the glory of God is revealed through the incorporation and healing of the sick and the outcast. Thus, to view the physical healing as an end in itself is to misinterpret the theological dynamic of the miracle and to impose an alien hermeneutical horizon. The most important outcome of the healing was not the physical healing but the leper's reconnection with God, self, and others, and the possibility that the community might become a faithful witness to the character and power of God as these things are made manifest in Jesus's physical healing of the leper.

None of this is to suggest that the physical healing of the leper was not important. Clearly the pain of leprosy is not to be desired. Jesus's healing is an embodiment and a revelation of God's love, compassion, grace, and healing power in the face of human suffering. Nevertheless, it is the suffering associated with the spiritual, theological, and communal dimensions of leprosy (isolation, exclusion, separation from God, meaninglessness) that is soul destroying and — when viewed through the lens of the hermeneutical perspective developed in this chapter — is the main target of the healing. The suffering that people with leprosy experienced within first-century Mediterranean culture transcended the boundaries of the physical pain or disfigurement of the pathological condition. If this is so, then the purpose and goal of the healing was primarily soteriological (aimed at reconnecting the individual with God), ecclesiological (designed to build up the people of God), and missiological (intended to show unbelievers the identity, nature, and personhood of Christ). The healing was an act of grace designed to reveal something of God and God's purposes for human beings.

But why send him to the temple? It could, of course, be argued that Jesus

healed the man and then sent him to the temple to be cleansed, the impli-
cation being that the social and theological significance of the temple rituals
that had initially served to oppress the man with leprosy remained in place,
thus excluding others with this condition. In other words, the man was healed,
but nothing really changed institutionally. However, this is not necessarily the
only interpretation we can draw. In touching and healing the leper, Jesus reconnected him with God. He then sent him to the temple. But, presumably,
he did not send him back to the temple to be cleansed and reconnected with
God; that had already been done via Jesus's healing touch. A more challenging
interpretation might be that, while Jesus sent him back to participate in the rituals of his religious community, the participation of the leper was intended to
transform the temple rituals rather than *conform* to them. The man approached
the temple rituals cleansed and assured of his relationship with God through
his encounter with Jesus. This being so, his participation in the temple rituals
had a different meaning from what was the assumed norm. His participation
was the following:

1. A profound witness *to* the priests; a testimony of who Jesus was and how
    God was to be accessed in the new kingdom. This was an important mis-
    siological move. If even the priests were satisfied with the healing, then
    Jesus's ministry would be validated from a very powerful social, political,
    and theological source.
2. A transformation of dimensions of the meaning of the rituals. Healing
    and reconnection with God were no longer necessarily tied to the temple
    alone. The temple rituals publicly symbolized the former leper's move-
    ment into the community, but not into the presence of God, as God was
    already with him. By sending the man to the temple, Jesus changed the
    meaning of the rituals into an act of validation and public welcoming. The
    rituals that once served as barriers to inclusion now became a testimony
    to Jesus.

Implications for the Understanding and Practice of Spiritual Healing

If we take on board the implications of the hermeneutical approach that has
been developed thus far, it is possible to develop a revised understanding of
spiritual healing that has considerable pastoral significance. The understanding presented here helps us pastorally in at least two ways. First, it offers some
critical insights into the nature, purpose, and goal of the contemporary healing

ministry and what might be appropriate and inappropriate expectations and goals. Second, it offers some fascinating possibilities for broadening our definition of spiritual healing and incorporating this into our pastoral practice. It will be helpful to examine both of these dimensions in turn.

Why are some healed and others not? A major ongoing debate within Christian healing today relates to this question. Spiritual healing within a Christian context is an act of grace that has a spiritual purpose that lies within and beyond the physical or psychological dimensions of the healing. The healing itself is an important act of divine compassion, but it must always be understood as a means to a greater end rather than an end in itself. This suggestion has important theological, pastoral, and ecclesiological implications. Despite the fact that some theologies of healing and the healing practices that emerge from them hold on to the possibility that spiritual healing functions according to the assumptions of the medical model and in line with the laws of cause and effect (enough faith = the certainty of healing), the reality for many people is that miraculous spiritual healing is sporadic and unpredictable. Standard responses to the sporadic nature of spiritual healing tend to hold on to the cause-and-effect dynamic and blame the persons who are not healed, accusing them of such things as a lack of faith, a failure to hold on to the correct Scripture, the presence of unforgiven sin in their lives, and so forth. Huge burdens of guilt are laid on people who, on most accounts, appear to be faithful but are not cured. The pastoral consequences of such understandings can be devastating. And yet God continues to cure people. How are we to understand and work with this tension?

If we follow through on the hermeneutical pattern that I have described in the earlier part of this chapter, we can begin to explore in a different way why some are healed and others are not. What I have suggested thus far is that Jesus's healings (and by definition the contemporary healings that are carried out in his name) should be understood theologically and recognized as eschatological signs or, as Ray Anderson puts it, "sacraments," through which the reality of the gospel promises are assured in a manner that is embodied and tangible. "The effect of the healing," Anderson continues, "is to strengthen faith in the reality of the resurrection and the forgiveness of sins, not to make faith dependent upon the effect of the healing itself."[19] Jesus's healings were public actions that affected not only the individual who was healed but also the entire community, calling both to more faithful forms of practice and a deeper relationship with God and with one another. Viewed in this way, the theological meaning of the

---

19. Ray S. Anderson, *Dancing with Wolves While Feeding the Sheep: Musings of a Maverick Theologian* (Eugene, OR: Wipf & Stock, 2002), 96.

miracle becomes liberatory for the healer, the one healed, and the community where the healing occurs. Such a perspective on spiritual healing liberates both those who are healed and those who are not healed. It frees those who are healed from the possible disappointment that they will get ill again in the future. The healed leper may well catch leprosy in the future. Physical and psychological healing is always temporary and transient; those who are healed today could easily become ill again tomorrow. However, if the healing is viewed primarily in terms of sacrament or revelation, the continuing potency of the healing is assured as is its place within the effective history of the community. In this sense, it is the community and not just the individual who is healed. This is so irrespective of the continuing health (or ill health) of the person who is healed. In other words, the meaning of the miracle continues to function soteriologically (in terms of affirming and encouraging salvation), well beyond the specific event of the physical action of healing. Indeed, the meaning of the healing may well change and develop as it embeds itself as part of the tradition and effective history of the community and develops its identity as a hermeneutical principle that people can use in times of sickness.

This way of understanding spiritual healing also has the effect of freeing persons who are not healed from the guilt or fear (if not from the disappointment) that not being healed is due to a lack of faith or a sign of divine displeasure. If healing is a gift of grace designed to encourage the faith and hope of the community and to draw people back to God, then *all* healings within the community should be viewed as opportunities to celebrate the affirmation that God is present and at work — even if, at that moment in time, particular individuals may not be the recipient of the healing. In this way, "the miracle of physical healing of a person considered as an eschatological sign of the resurrection delivers the church from the temptation to set up physical healing as a special sign of God's grace for those who have sufficient faith. The church is thus delivered from the tendency to make out of physical healing a manipulation of faith and a pragmatic method by which the growth of the church can be assured. That which has the character of a sacrament is an eschatological event and can never be subject to control or manipulation."[20] Such a liberating perspective not only emphasizes the ultimate significance of spiritual healing but also offers a powerful critique of approaches to healing that understand the healing as an end in itself, rather than as a way of accessing that which transcends the physical and psychological dimensions of the healing process.

20. Anderson, *Dancing with Wolves*, 96.

Spiritual Healing as Reinterpretation and Reconnection: The Case of Severe Mental Health Challenges

Thus far I have used the term *spiritual healing* to refer to healing that occurs via a direct supernatural intervention from God that impacts individuals and communities in profound ways. However, the discussion on the significance of the meaning of such healing, particularly as it relates to a highly stigmatized condition such as leprosy, has raised some potentially vital pastoral perspectives that allow us to consider spiritual healing within a broader framework of Christian healing, one that includes but is not defined by direct divine intervention. In light of the previous discussion, it is possible to develop a working definition of Christian healing as relating to the development of *forms of thought, action, and relationship carried out in the name of Jesus, which lead to the reframing of the experience and understanding of disease in ways that bring about positive relationships with God, others, and with one's self.* Such thought, action, and relationship function primarily to reconnect individuals and communities with God, quite apart from the presence or absence of particular forms of pathology or outcomes that are determined by the presence or absence of a cure. Healing, then, is not dependent on the *absence* of disease but rather on the *presence* of certain forms of relationship that lead to the renegotiation of the meanings of physical or psychological disease. This process of renegotiating meanings and the living out of these new meanings forms the essence of a holistic view of Christian healing that includes but is not defined by the supernatural.

Spirituality and Severe Mental Health Challenges

We have seen that a primary meaning of the gospel miracles relates to *reinterpretation* and *reconnection*; the reinterpretation of human experience in the light of a new divine hermeneutic and the reconnection and reorientation of persons who have been dislocated from God, self, others, and community. A useful way of drawing the previous discussion into a contemporary pastoral context is through a brief examination of how the understanding presented in this chapter might relate to the lives of people with severe mental health challenges. As we shall see, there are some fascinating parallels between the contemporary experience of this group of people, those suffering from leprosy in Jesus's time, and the practical theological response that Jesus made to the leper in the passage we looked at previously. Drawing out some of these parallels will enable us to begin to see how the ideas laid out in this chapter might help as we seek to offer pastoral care that is faithful and healing.

The situation of people with severe mental health challenges within Western cultures is often a profoundly negative one. People with this experience find that their lives are marred by stigma, depersonalization, social, relational, spiritual, and political exclusion, physical and sexual abuse, and hopelessness.[21] In a very real sense, they are a group of people who, like "Jesus's leper," have been forced onto the margins of society. The horizon of Western culture has deeply ingrained prejudices relating to the primacy of the rational. (I use the term *prejudice* here in its pejorative sense.) As Stephen Post correctly observes, "we live in a culture that is the child of rationalism and capitalism, so clarity of mind and economic productivity determine the value of a human life."[22] Within such a culture, those who appear to be losing these qualities are always vulnerable to abuse and exclusion. To have a mental health challenge can be a deeply dehumanizing experience insofar as such things as reason and clarity of mind are often deeply tied in with what many presume to be the essence of humanness. It would not be an exaggeration to describe people with severe mental health challenges as "modern day lepers."[23] Ironically, in light of the story we explored above, Christian communities can be as isolating and stigmatizing as any other aspect of society, in both their theology and their practices.[24]

It is interesting to notice that the name of the leper in the story of Jesus's healing is not given. He is defined by his disease. This omission resonates closely with the experiences of many people with severe mental health challenges, which tend to be totalizing entities. By this I mean that, unlike those with the measles, influenza, or appendicitis, people *become* their illnesses. People do not become the flu or the measles, but they do become schizophrenics or manic depressives. This enforced negative identity has a profound impact on their life trajectories and experiences. The diagnosis of a severe mental health challenge such as schizophrenia or bipolar disorder forms a cultural horizon (in the Gadamerian sense) that totally subsumes the person to his or her diagnosis: body, mind, and soul. Within such a cultural context, all the actions and experiences of the person with the mental health challenge, including his or her expressions of spirituality, tend to be interpreted through the lens of pathology. God becomes

21. For a deeper exploration of this point, see my *Resurrecting the Person: Friendship and the Care of Those Suffering with Mental Health Problems* (Nashville: Abingdon, 2000).

22. Stephen G. Post, *The Moral Challenge of Alzheimer Disease* (Baltimore: Johns Hopkins University Press, 1995), 3.

23. B. Johnson, "Modern Day Lepers," in *Personality Disorder and Human Worth: Papers from a Conference Organised by the Board of Social Responsibility* (London: The Church of England Board of Social Responsibility, 2002), 13–20.

24. For more on this point, see Swinton, *Resurrecting the Person*.

nothing but a pathological dimension of his or her experience. People cannot worship God, because God is inevitably perceived as a delusion. In other words, there is often an inherent prejudice (both in the Gadamerian sense and in the more pejorative sense) built on false perceptions of the spiritual lives of people with severe mental health challenges that serves to firmly close the temple gates from the inside (their experience is assumed to be false or distorted) and from the outside (Christian communities tend to shy away from unusual behavior and experience, hence the lack of welcome for people with severe mental health challenges). Despite the fact that many people with severe mental health challenges have significant spiritual needs and are clear that they want churches and established mental health services to meet these needs, their spirituality continues to be problematic for psychiatry and church alike.[25] When persons, as mental patients, have their spiritual voice removed, crucial dimensions of these persons, as persons, are lost. They find themselves, in a real sense, excluded from the temple — that is, those services, relationships, ways of thinking, and practices that people require in order to hold on to God in the midst of their deepest storms. What, then, might the idea of spiritual healing as reinterpretation and reconnection mean for people with this kind of experience?

Religion and Mental Health

If healing has to do with the renegotiation of meanings and the reconnection of persons with God, self, and others, then the place to begin to think about what healing might look like in the context of severe mental health challenge will be to explore whether the basic premise of the standard explanatory discussion is in fact accurate. Put slightly differently, if the horizon within which many mental health professionals and religious communities function in relation to severe mental

25. One survey estimated that 75 percent of British psychiatrists do not believe in God. See J. Neeleman and M. King, "Psychiatrists' Religious Attitudes in Relation to Their Clinical Practice: A Survey of 231 Psychiatrists," *Acta Psychiatrica Scandinavica* 88 (1994): 420–24. Bergin and Jensen found that a similarly high proportion of American psychotherapists had little or no spiritual affiliation. See A. E. Bergin and J. P. Jensen, "Religiosity of Psychotherapists: A National Survey," *Psychotherapy* 27 (1990): 3–7. This contrasts significantly with the Mental Health Foundation's more recent work (*Taken Seriously: The Somerset Spirituality Project* [London: Mental Health Foundation, 2002]), which showed clearly that the service users who took part in the study held religious or spiritual beliefs — which they viewed as important in helping them cope with their mental health challenges — and highlighted the need for encouragement in discussing such concerns with mental health care workers.

health challenges and religious belief is inaccurate, then the role of religion and religious communities will necessarily shift in response. Like Jesus touching the leper, such a shift may become the locus for reframing and healing.

One of the questions that is frequently asked in relation to religion and severe mental health challenges relates to the issue of causality: Does religion *cause* mental health challenges (in particular, psychosis)? Indeed, an assumed affirmative answer to this question has proven to be a major barrier in incorporating issues of religion into contemporary psychiatric practices. The argument goes something like this: People with severe mental health challenges frequently express their illness experiences through religious delusions and hallucinations; *therefore*, religion cannot be a good thing, as it "obviously" feeds the pathology and often produces anxiety and an exacerbation of the patient's condition. This being so, "in the interest of the patient," religion should be excluded from the therapeutic process. It is certainly true that religion is a powerful epistemological force that can be difficult and sometimes dangerous in a mental health context, as it can in any context. Care, sensitivity, and thoughtfulness are required, combined with continuing dialogue between experts in psychological care and experts in religious and spiritual care, such as hospital chaplains.[26] However, the difficulties that religion poses do not necessitate its exclusion. Accepted practices such as psychopharmacology or electroconvulsive therapy can also be very dangerous and destructive if they are misused. The key is to integrate attention to religion in a way that allows constructive and protective dialogue around the key issues as they emerge. But beyond this, one has to ask whether the assumption that religion is causally implicated in severe mental health challenges is in fact the case, or whether in fact it is our prejudices and the limitations of the psychiatric horizon (a horizon that powerfully shapes other cultural horizons) that make this *appear* to be the case? Could the ways we think about the relationship between severe mental health challenges and religion actually be a symptom of the mental health challenge — that is, a pathological aspect of the person's condition that causes and adds to their anxiety, distress, alienation, and isolation? In other words, could it be that current framings of severe mental health challenges actually cause a form of "leprosy" that blocks people from accessing God?

The Hermeneutics of Mental Health Challenges

In an important paper exploring the hermeneutics of religion and mental health, Williams and Faulconer present an argument for the reinterpretation of the ex-

---

26. For a deeper discussion around this issue, see my *Spirituality and Mental Health Care*.

pression of spiritual experience within psychotic illnesses. They highlight the modernist roots of psychiatry's understanding of the role of religion within mental health challenges and offer a critique of the cause-and-effect dynamics of the medical model. In particular, they are critical of this assumption: "For every disorder there is a pathogen, some substance or set of substances, which causes disorder, and the recovery of the pathogen is a sufficient explanation of the disorder."[27] Within this approach, mental health challenges are seen as analogous to physical illnesses in that they comprise a fixed chain of cause-and-effect events running from *pathogen* to *symptom* to *diagnosis* to *treatment* to *cure*. Williams and Faulconer argue that the problem with this approach is that it is fundamentally reductionist in that it "translates the phenomena it observes into its own narrower terms of analysis. Psychology reduces phenomena to the language of efficient causation" (338). So religious experience is inevitably translated into its presumed psychological equivalent. The problem is that it is not easy, if indeed possible, to translate the language of religion into the language of psychology. The language of cross, resurrection, and sin simply do not have psychological equivalents.

In response to this situation, Williams and Faulconer offer a hermeneutical alternative that takes seriously the lived experiences of religion and spirituality within the context of severe mental health challenges. Rather than simply reducing the expression of spiritual experiences to pathology and assuming them to be *nothing but* a causal dimension of a person's illness, they argue that it is necessary to explore what religious and spiritual experiences are as discrete personal events that should be understood in and of themselves, not simply in relation to a person's pathology. Within this perspective, religious experience is not viewed as a variable but as a *language* that gives to both participant and observer a perspective and an account of their world — a horizon. Importantly, they remark, "Psychopathology is viewed, not as an end state following necessarily from causal chains of events and conditions, but as an interpretive act which discloses the way or manner of one's situatedness in the social world. Psychopathology is an 'expression' of one's situation, an expression necessarily occurring in some form of language" (339). Rather than being *nothing but* pathology, within this reframing of illness, the expression of religious and spiritual experience — conveyed through religious language — becomes a significant expression of a person's lifeworld, which requires interpretation and understanding. "Physiological or other powerful conditions in the life of any person may function as part, even a major part,

27. Richard Williams and James Faulconer, "Religion and Mental Health: A Hermeneutical Reconsideration," *Review of Religious Research* 35, no. 4 (June 1994): 336. Hereafter, in this section, page references will be given in parentheses in the text.

of any psychological pathology. The pathology itself, however, is always more than these conditions — it is the agent's expression of her condition, including the physical, in whatever way she is able to express it — in other words, using whatever language and elements of expression she has available" (340). Religious and spiritual experience is thus understood as a form of language that people use to express their experiences in a way that encapsulates the things that are most significant to them. It may well be affected by the symptoms of the person's particular mental health challenge, but it cannot be defined by or reduced to such, any more than so-called nonreligious psychotic expression is indicative that there is no nonreligious world "out there." Bearing in mind that religious language expresses that which is deepest and most significant for persons on a temporal and a transcendent level, it is only natural that people with severe mental health challenges will communicate their experiences in the language that is most deeply significant for them. "Therefore," Williams and Faulconer continue, "even when the tensions faced by those people are not specifically religious tensions, we should not be surprised to find them expressed in religious language" (340). Importantly, as mentioned above, if misinterpreted, this spiritual language may well *not* translate into the language of psychiatry in ways other than through the negative horizon of pathology. The language of sin, cross, salvation, and redemption does not fit well into horizons that give primacy to the significance of diagnostic criteria and scientific validity over lived experience. In the same way the religious people of Jesus's time did not have a broad enough linguistic horizon to understand what Jesus was doing and to create a space for lepers, the language and horizon of mental health professionals may well be too narrow to encompass the fullness of patients' experiences and the true nature of their healing.

None of this is to suggest that mental health challenges are not real or that there is no need for psychiatric intervention. My argument is for the merging of the psychiatric and the spiritual horizons, not the eradication of one or the other. Nevertheless, unless the horizon of the mental health care provider can effectively and respectfully merge with the spiritual horizon of the sufferer, mental health care will always deal only with a part of the person, to the neglect of the whole. Healing will always and inevitably be limited.

Christian Healing as Reinterpreting, Translating, Dialoguing, and Understanding

If this analysis is correct, then healing within the context of severe mental health challenges relates to much more than simply eradicating or controlling an individual's pathology (although it may well include actions designed to do this, both divine and temporal). Indeed, the eradication of pathology would not necessarily overcome the stigma, exclusion, and disconnection that people with severe mental health challenges experience.[28] Being cured of a mental health challenge can often lead to the creation of new identity — an ex-mental patient — wherein the stigma, exclusion, and isolation associated with mental health challenges continue within the social arena even though it has found its resolution within the psychological.[29] Christian healing within this context relates to *reinterpreting* a person's situation (in word and deed, finding ways of moving her from mental patient to person), recognizing her significance as a spiritual being and striving to understand and respect the spiritual language that she is using to communicate her experiences and her desire to reach for God. Healing then relates to the ability of carers to *understand* the meaning of a person's spiritual expressions without trying to *translate* them into a different language. This means moving beyond the negative horizons that are created by diagnoses and cultural assumptions and finding a space to be with the person with a mental health challenge in a way that not only respects her language and experience but is also prepared to learn from it.

Such a reframing of healing proposes that religion and spirituality can heal but not necessarily in the way that the medical model suggests healing should be understood. Williams and Faulconer put this point in this way:

> Can religion heal, or has it rightly forfeited that function to psychology? The answer to this question revolves around what we take healing to be. If, as the modern psychological perspective, healing is a mainly technological function best modelled on medical science, if healing is intervention in a causal chain, then it is best left to the technologists, and the efficient causal model will suffice. In fact, if the modernist perspective is right, the medical causal model is necessary to legitimate our healing technologies. However, if psychological pathology is a moral problem — where any problem occurring in a social, historical world is necessarily moral in the broad sense — then healing is a moral activity, involving the reconciliation of people and worlds rather than causal intervention. If psychopathology is a moral problem, then

---

28. It is important to bear in mind here that the removal of the pathology would not necessarily remove the problem for the person; it would simply move him or her from a mental patient to an ex-mental patient. The exclusion, stigma, and alienation are not necessarily altered by miraculous healing of the condition. Healing can come only when the meanings of the condition are renegotiated and reframed within the community.

29. See, for example, Peter Barham and Robert Hayward, *Relocating Madness: From the Mental Patient to the Person* (New York: New York University Press, 1995).

healing is therapy in its root sense, the work of a servant rather than, as in empiricistic psychology, the work of a trained mechanic.[30]

Healing then has to do with recovering forgotten meanings and enabling the possibility of giving voice to those dimensions of human experience that are fundamental to the lived experience of persons but have been occluded by the volume of the voices of the medical model.

Conclusion: Healing as Mediation and Interpretation

Christian healing occurs when the followers of Jesus begin to work with these assumptions and seek, in a variety of ways, to facilitate — via the kinds of practical hermeneutical approaches outlined in this chapter — the reconnection of people with God, self, and others. This means, *inter alia*, challenging the established sources of interpretive authority (psychiatric and ecclesial) that have the social, political, and spiritual power to validate or invalidate particular experiences and forms of language. In the same way that Jesus's touching of the leper challenged the community to rethink its values and boundaries, challenging established forms of knowledge and assumptions that might block a person's passage to God is a key healing task. The case of severe mental health challenges helps illustrate and make this case. Within a hospital context, such a challenge can come from, for example, a mental health chaplain who is called to be both a prophetic witness on behalf of a different horizon and the mediator between the psychiatric and the spiritual horizons. By embodying the horizon of the spiritual in his or her caring encounters with both sufferers and those who seek to offer care and support to them, the chaplain can initiate transforming conversations that will lead to a new merging of horizons that takes seriously the need to listen to the language of the spiritual and offer effective and meaningful spiritual care. In renegotiating the meaning of the experiences of people with severe mental health challenges, the chaplain (or any other Christian interpreter) begins to initiate the types of healing that we discover in the ministry of Jesus. Many current attitudes tend, as it were, to exclude people with severe mental health challenges from the temple — that is, to deny them access to conversations and perspectives that might help them maintain their relationship with God, self, and others even in the midst of the most troublesome storms. The presence of the chaplain within the system of care ensures that invalidated

30. Williams and Faulconer, "Religion and Mental Health," 345.

experiences are revalidated and that established interpretations of the experience of severe mental health challenges are not allowed to militate against the possibility of healing and spiritual reinterpretation and reincorporation. What is true for the chaplain as representative of the church is also true for the whole church. The church is called to be an interpretative community, a place where the outcast can find a spiritual home.[31]

It is clear, then, that Christian healing is a much broader and more complex concept than it is often assumed to be. It involves both spiritual healing, which is marked by God's direct intervention, and Christian healing, which is the wider ministry carried out by Christians. This latter mode of healing focuses on the same theological principles as does spiritual healing, but its approaches do not necessarily require intervention that is directly supernatural. The perspective on spiritual healing offered here opens up the concept to include wider interpersonal, hermeneutical, social, and communal dimensions. The implications of our reflections on spirituality within mental health challenges suggest that healing is not the task of the lone healer but the work of communities (secular and religious) who recognize the need to reframe their understandings of human well-being in light of those who are being excluded as a result of current forms of understanding and practice. Certainly physical and psychological healing will remain a significant dimension of our understanding of spiritual healing. However, perhaps more important are the other dimensions that explore the ways people who have become marginalized and dislocated from the community can be "touched," depolluted, and effectively reincorporated into the community, a place where they can experience meaningful relationships with God, self, and others. This is the way to peace, the way of *shalom*.

31. For a full account of how this might be possible, see my *Resurrecting the Person*, esp. chs. 9–11.

Conclusion

Whither Spiritual Healing Now?

Sarah Coakley

Ａt the end of his remarkable book *Being Mortal: Illness, Medicine, and What Matters in the End*, the Harvard surgeon and medical writer Atul Gawande recounts the story of scattering his father's ashes over the waters of the Ganges, according to the instructions left to him.[1] As he records in intricate detail the Hindu religious rituals involved in the event (the services of a *pandit* — a holy man — had been secured in advance), one is aware of the complexity of Gawande's own emotions of grief in a context of religious meaning, from which he is now himself personally removed — by geography as well as by conviction. It had fallen to Gawande to assist his father in another way at the end, as a secularized doctor in North America unusually unafraid to acknowledge the limits of life and so to speak the truth about when it was time to stop treatment in the face of the inevitable. But in telling the story of the later visit to the Ganges, he movingly acknowledges the strangely *healing* nature of the religious rites that his father had insisted upon: "Floating on that swollen river, I could not help sensing the hands of the many generations connected across time. In bringing us there, my father had helped us see that he was part of a story going back thousands of years — and so were we."[2] In this meaning-making event, artfully predetermined by his father, Gawande's grief is mysteriously assuaged.

As I wrote in the introduction to this book, "In the context of the Western cultural contradictions over health and suffering . . . , the phenomenon of spir-

---

1. Atul Gawande, *Being Mortal: Illness, Medicine, and What Matters in the End* (London: Profile, 2015).

2. Gawande, *Being Mortal*, 262.

itual healing is at base a manifestation that calls forth a world of *value*."[3] Gawande's narrative is a particularly poignant example of this truth, combining — in his case — religious eclecticism, metaphysical doubt, scientific realism, and moral discernment. There are indeed infinite varieties of such a combination of discrete elements in the quest for healing in the face of suffering and death.

Overall, then, this book has been devoted to clarifying how science, medicine, ritual, metaphysics, theology, hermeneutics, moral theory, and pastoral caregiving are all conjoined and intermingled in the phenomenon we have come to call spiritual healing. As it happens, this volume is for me — as editor and theologian — the third and last in a trilogy of interdisciplinary volumes that have investigated from various methodological directions the body and its multiple meanings;[4] but this last one on healing has involved far and away the most complex and intricate analysis of interdisciplinary convergences on a phenomenon still necessarily shrouded in a degree of mystery, even of transcendent allure. Let me just recapitulate in closing why this is so and what this may mean for future and further creative research on the topic of spiritual healing. I shall make only three brief points.

First, I must say something about the ongoing debates between science and religion and what this volume has taught us in relation to spiritual healing. The contributors to this book have raised profound and searching questions about the *inadvisability* of trying to probe the veracity of spiritual healing via medical prayer studies that seek to isolate the God element, simplistically, in clinical outcomes. If nothing else has been learned from this book, it should be that the complex relations of science and religion in the area of spiritual healing must, perforce, involve subtler negotiations of the relevant disciplines and methodological presumptions than has yet been acknowledged. But this does not mean that the task is impossible; much is still to be done. Thick descriptions of healing events (such as the sensitive anthropological studies we have seen in this volume) are crucial for charting the human *experience* of healing; and metaphysical discussion-points about the presumptions of scientific naturalism and its limitations are just as important as empirical studies in this area of debate. In short, there will be no solution to the science-versus-religion debate in relation to spiritual healing without bringing in the other disciplines with which this book has consistently engaged. The interdisciplinary task must go on.

Second, when we come to reflect on the *theological* options for explaining

3. See p. 26, above.

4. The two earlier books were mentioned also in the introduction: Sarah Coakley, ed., *Religion and the Body* (Cambridge: Cambridge University Press, 1997), and Sarah Coakley and Kay Kaufman Shelemay, eds., *Pain and Its Transformations: The Interface of Biology and Culture* (Cambridge, MA: Harvard University Press, 2007).

spiritual healing, this book has proposed a number of metaphysical possibilities that also require ongoing reflection and adjudication. Indeed, we have rehearsed a number of different religious and philosophical accounts of spiritual healing in this volume; each has its own rationality and cogency, and each requires further consideration and investigation. The lesson to be learned here is that the choice between these various possibilities is not just an optional dimension of reflection on healing but also demands further critical debate and discernment. In particular, those engaged in healing practices in parish life *ought* to be thinking deeply about the biblical, theological, and philosophical issues that their undertakings evoke and enshrine, and how they relate to quite practical insights and outcomes. That does not mean, of course, that such lessons will be directly conveyed to those in need of healing in the midst of a service or rite; but it does mean that the healing ministry is at some level necessarily informed by such philosophical and theological reflection, and from there linked to the crucial nexus of faith, hope, and love inherent in all aspirations to healing.

Third and finally, then, the *pastoral* implications of the contents of this volume are concomitantly various and far-reaching. What has been urged throughout this volume is that meaning-making is all-important in the matter of healing: the quest for a narrative of purpose and resolution attends all and every human experience of pain and suffering (whether spoken or unspoken). The primary role of the minister or caregiver is thus attentively to stand alongside those who seek such a meaning-making, without forcing the outcome or preordaining the result. Indeed, at the end of life when words fail, and meaning often seems elusive or even absent, it is the particular role of the minister or family member simply to *witness* to the mystery of what is occurring, without judgment or intervention. This in itself is a spiritual exercise of great demand, discipline, and honor. Only later — sometimes much later — does the meaning of what has happened and its healing potential become fully apparent.

This book has been edited and produced in the conviction that spiritual healing (in both of the senses described in the introduction) does indeed happen and that the expectation of such is not only not unreasonable but also positively to be hoped and prayed for. For those more skeptical about the matter, however, there is also plenty in this volume to fuel their reflective instincts and further incite the philosophical and scientific debates that this book has attempted to sharpen and clarify. The debate must go on.

Acknowledgments

The editor is glad to acknowledge gratitude to a number of institutions and people who have made the production of this book possible and aided its path to publication.

First and most importantly, the volume owes its inception to a symposium on spiritual healing, generously funded by the Templeton Foundation under the Humble Approach Initiative, and most ably and energetically supported by Dr. Mary Ann Meyers, senior fellow at the foundation. Without her initiative and insight, neither the original conference nor the scholarly products that have emerged from it would have taken the shape and substance that they have. Indeed, such was the stimulation of the original meeting, that it was decided after it that each of the co-convenors — Dr. Fraser Watts (then of Cambridge University) and myself — would edit volumes with slightly different emphases and focuses of interest, since the complexity and import of the conference material clearly merited this path. Dr. Meyers's guidance, and the further financial support of the Templeton Foundation, was particularly helpful at this juncture of decision. Dr. Watts's edited volume appeared first under the title *Spiritual Healing: Scientific and Religious Perspectives* (Cambridge University Press, 2014) and made direct divine action and the psychology of healing central to its reflection. This current volume, while rehearsing afresh the definitions of spiritual healing forged at the original symposium, has found its core interest in the hermeneutics and meaning-making involved in spiritual healing, the relation of that factor to contemporary neuroscience and clinical practice, and the importance of the theological category of secondary causation for the topic of healing.

I must also take this opportunity to express my personal gratitude to the Leverhulme Foundation and to the McDonald Agape Foundation, both of which have generously funded my own scholarly work during the period this book has been completed.

The substantial undertaking of editing this book could not have been completed without the meticulous and dedicated work of three junior colleagues who have assisted me at Harvard University and at the University of Cambridge, as doctoral or postdoctoral students: Drs. Zachary Simpson, Samuel Hole, and Emily S. Kempson. Their assistance has been invaluable.

Finally, I must express my gratitude to those at Eerdmans who have supported this project from the start: Bill Eerdmans himself, Jon Pott, and (more recently) James Ernest and his team. Their patience and professionalism are, in equal measure, remarkable, and I give them due thanks.

— *Sarah Coakley*

Contributors

Emma Anderson is professor in the Department of Classics and Religious Studies at the University of Ottawa. She is the author of two books published by Harvard University Press, *The Betrayal of Faith: The Tragic Journey of a Colonial Native Convert* (2007) and *The Death and Afterlife of the North American Martyrs* (2013), as well as numerous chapters in edited volumes and articles in academic journals.

Stephen R. L. Clark is emeritus professor of philosophy at the University of Liverpool and an honorary research fellow in the Department of Theology at the University of Bristol. His books include *From Athens to Jerusalem* (1984, 2019), *A Parliament of Souls* (1990), *God, Religion and Reality* (1998), *G. K. Chesterton: Thinking Backwards, Looking Forwards* (2006), *Understanding Faith* (2009), *Ancient Mediterranean Philosophy* (2013), *Plotinus: Myth, Metaphor and Philosophical Practice* (2016), and *Can We Believe in People?* (2020). His chief current interests are in the philosophy of Plotinus, the understanding and treatment of nonhuman animals, the philosophy of religion, and science fiction.

Philip Clayton is the Ingraham Professor of Theology at Claremont School of Theology. Before joining the faculty at CST, Dr. Clayton taught or held research professorships at Williams College, the California State University, Harvard University, Cambridge University, and the University of Munich. Dr. Clayton is a constructive Christian theologian, deeply engaged in dialogue with science, contemporary philosophy, and the world's religious traditions. He has authored or edited twenty-four books, including (with Steven Knapp) *The Predicament of Belief: Science, Philosophy, Faith* (2011), *Religion and Science: The Basics*

(2011), *Adventures in the Spirit* (2009), *Transforming Christian Theology* (2009), *In Quest of Freedom* (2009), (coeditor) *Evolution and Ethics: Human Morality in Biological and Religious Perspective* (2006), and (editor) *The Oxford Handbook of Religion and Science* (2006). Earlier books include (coeditor) *Science and the Spiritual Quest* (2002), *God and Contemporary Science* (1997), and *The Problem of God in Modern Thought* (2000).

Sarah Coakley is Norris-Hulse Professor Emerita at the University of Cambridge, honorary professor at the Logos Institute, University of St. Andrews, honorary fellow, Oriel College, Oxford, and professorial research fellow at the Institute of Religion and Critical Inquiry, Australian Catholic University, Melbourne and Rome. In 2019 she was elected a fellow of the British Academy. A systematic theologian and philosopher of religion who has wide interdisciplinary interests, her publications relevant to this volume include (editor) *Religion and the Body* (1997), *Powers and Submissions: Spirituality, Philosophy and Gender* (2002), (coeditor) *Pain and Its Transformations* (2007), (coeditor) *Evolution, Games and God* (2013), *God, Sexuality and the Self: An Essay 'On the Trinity'* (2013), and *The New Asceticism: Sexuality, Gender and the Quest for God* (2015). Her Gifford Lectures on evolutionary cooperation are soon to be published and are available online at https://www.giffordlectures.org/lectures /sacrifice-regained-evolution-cooperation-and-god.

Thomas J. Csordas is the Dr. James Y. Chan Presidential Chair in Global Health, professor and chair in the Department of Anthropology, director of the Global Health Program, and codirector of the Global Health Institute at the University of California, San Diego. He is also a member of the American Society for the Study of Religion and former president of the Society for the Anthropology of Religion. Among his publications are *The Sacred Self: A Cultural Phenomenology of Charismatic Healing* (1994), (editor) *Embodiment and Experience: The Existential Ground of Culture and Self* (1994), *Language, Charisma, and Creativity: Ritual Life in the Catholic Charismatic Renewal* (1997), *Body/Meaning/Healing* (2002), and (editor) *Transnational Transcendence: Essays on Religion and Globalization* (2009).

Heather D. Curtis is professor of religion at Tufts University, where she also holds appointments in the Department of Studies in Race, Colonialism, and Diaspora; the Department of History; and the International Relations programs. Curtis received her doctorate in the history of Christianity and American religion from Harvard University. She is the author of *Faith in the Great Physician: Suffering and Divine Healing in American Culture, 1860–1900* (2007), which was awarded the Frank S. and Elizabeth D. Brewer prize from the American Society of Church History for the best first book in the history of Christianity. Her most recent book, *Holy Humanitarians: American Evangelicals and Global Aid* (2018), examines the crucial role evangelical missionaries and popular religious media played in the extension of US aid at home and abroad from the late nineteenth to the early twentieth century. Curtis is currently at work on a religious biography of Ida B. Wells for the Oxford University Spiritual Lives series.

Howard L. Fields is professor emeritus of neurology and former director of the Wheeler Center for the Neurobiology of Addiction at the University of California, San Francisco. He is a distinguished scientist and physician with expertise in the area of pain and drug addiction, with a focus on nervous system mechanisms and how endogenous opioids contribute to these mechanisms. He received his MD and PhD in Neuroscience at Stanford in 1965–66 and trained in clinical neurology at Harvard. He was a founder of the UCSF Pain Management Center and has made major contributions to understanding and treating neuropathic pain. He has over three hundred scientific publications and has received numerous research awards. His influential monograph, *Pain* (1987), was translated into Italian, French, and Japanese. His honors include a Merit Award from the NIH, the Kerr Award of the American Pain Society, the Cotzias Award of the American Academy of Neurology and the R. D. Adams lecture of the American Neurological Association, and the Founder's Award from the American Academy of Pain Medicine. He has also given the Beecher Lecture and the Adams Lecture at Harvard. He is an elected member of the Institute of Medicine (1997) and the American Academy of Arts and Sciences (2010).

Beverly Roberts Gaventa is Distinguished Professor of New Testament at Baylor University and Helen H. P. Manson Professor of New Testament Literature Emerita at Princeton Theological Seminary. She has been active in a number of professional societies, including Studiorum Novi Testamenti Societas, the Society of Biblical Literature (of which she was president in 2016), and the American Theological Association. She has served on a number of editorial boards and lectured widely in the United States, Canada, Europe, South Africa, and Australia. In addition to numerous articles and edited volumes, she is the author of *From Darkness to Light: Aspects of Conversion in the New Testament* (1986), *I and II Thessalonians* (1998), *Mary: Glimpses of the Mother of Jesus* (1999), *The Acts of the Apostles* (2003), *Our Mother Saint Paul* (2007), and *When in Romans: An Invitation to Linger with the Gospel according to Paul* (2016).

Anne Harrington is the Franklin L. Ford Professor of the History of Science at Harvard University and director of Undergraduate Studies, specializing in the history of psychiatry, neuroscience, and the other mind and behavioral sciences. For six years she codirected Harvard's Mind, Brain, and Behavior Initiative. She was a consultant for the MacArthur Foundation Research Network on Mind-Body Interaction, and also served for twelve years on the Board of the Mind and Life Institute, dedicated to cross-cultural exchange and collaboration between the sciences and various contemplative traditions. She was a founding coeditor of *Biosocieties*, a journal concerned with social-science approaches to the life sciences. Professor Harrington is the author of three books: *Medicine, Mind and the Double Brain* (1987), *Reenchanted Science* (1997), and *The Cure Within: A History of Mind-Body Medicine* (2007). She is currently completing a new book, tentatively titled *The Biological Revolution in Psychiatry: What Really Happened?* Recent articles and chapters include "Zen, Suzuki, and the Art of Psychotherapy" (2016), "Mother Love and Mental Illness: An Emotional History" (2016), and "When Mindfulness Is Therapy" (2015). She is also developing a new research project on the history of "miracle healings" at the Catholic healing shrine of Lourdes.

Malcolm Jeeves, CBE, a past president of the Royal Society of Edinburgh (Scotland's National Academy) and former editor-in-chief of *Neuropsychologia*, is professor emeritus of psychology at the University of St. Andrews. He was Foundation Professor of Psychology there for twenty-four years and established the university's acclaimed psychology department. His own research has focused on brain mechanisms and neuroplasticity. He has authored sixteen books, including ten related to science and faith, and his studies particularly relevant to this volume are *Human Nature at the Millennium* (1997), (with R. J. Berry) *Science, Life, and Christian Belief* (1998), (with Warren Brown) *Neuroscience, Psychology, and Religion: Illusions, Delusions, and Realities about Human Nature* (2009), and *Minds, Brains, Souls, and Gods: A Conversation on Faith, Psychology, and Neuroscience* (2013). He has also edited several volumes of essays: *From Cells to Souls — and Beyond: Changing Portraits of Human Nature* (2004), *Rethinking Human Nature* (2011), and *The Emergence of Personhood: A Quantum Leap?* (2015). All of these last are published by Eerdmans.

John Swinton is professor in practical theology and pastoral care at the University of Aberdeen and master of Christ's College, Aberdeen. He is also honorary professor of nursing at Aberdeen University's Centre for Advanced Studies in Ministry. Professor Swinton is an ordained minister of the Church of Scotland,

and he worked as a registered nurse specializing in psychiatry and learning disabilities before becoming a community health chaplain. In 2004, he founded and is now director of the University of Aberdeen's Centre for Spirituality, Health and Disability (http://www.abdn.ac.uk/sdhp/centre-for-spirituality -health-and-disability-182.php). His work — focusing on the relationship between spirituality, theology, and health and the theology of disability — has been funded by the British Academy, the Arts and Humanities Research Council, the John Templeton Foundation, the Scottish Government, the Department of Health, the Mental Health Foundation, and the Foundation for People with Learning Disabilities (FPLD). He has published widely in his major fields of interest. His publications include *Becoming Friends of Time: Disability, Timefullness, and Gentle Discipleship* (2016), *Dementia: Living in the Memories of God* (2012), (with Brian Brock) *Disability in the Christian Tradition* (2012), *Raging with Compassion: Pastoral Responses to the Problem of Evil* (2007), and *Spirituality in Mental Health Care: Rediscovering a "Forgotten" Dimension* (2001).

Index of Authors

Index of Subjects

alternative therapies, 7, 12, 30, 155
Alzheimer's disease: and spiritual
experience, 102–3, 113–14, 155
anthropology, 10, 13n30, 16–17, 138,
139, 144, 183–84, 203–4; accounts of
spiritual healing, 186–92, 194–200
Aquinas, Thomas, 19–20, 21–22
Augustine, 159, 167–68, 171n36, 179

Baxter, Elizabeth, 67
belief (religious): embodied/embed-
ded nature of, 99, 100–101, 112–14;
and health benefits, 114–16, 119–21;
rationality of, 18–23; role in spiritual
healing, 12, 14–15, 48–50, 57, 88, 89,
90–92, 93, 97, 140, 144–45, 223n25;
significance of, 78, 81, 82–83, 103
Bernheim, Hippolyte, 122–23
biblical perspectives on healing, 29–39,
213–14, 216–18
biomedicine, 7, 10–16, 54–56, 211–16,
227–28
Boardman, William E., 66
brain: and behavior, 104–5, 108; function of, 88–90, 99–100, 102, 105–6,

107; influence on body, 10–11, 92,
93–97, 123–24; relationship to mind,
115, 136, 146, 151–52. *See also* mind-
brain relationship
Buckley, James M., 75

Catholic Church: and charismatic spiritual healing, 183, 184, 185–90, 201;
definitions of miraculous healing,
54–56; response to Marian appari-
tions/healings, 17, 41, 51–53, 57–58,
121–22
Charcot, Jean-Martin, 122, 123
Christian Science, 17, 18, 60–61;
critiques of, 73–77; development of,
64–66; and faith cure, 63–64, 68–69;
vs. naturalism/skepticism, 72–73,
77–78, 81; and practice of prayer,
78–81
cognitive processes: embodied nature,
100–101, 108–9, 110–11; and neural
systems, 102, 104, 106–7
community: and healing in Scripture, 20–21, 34–36, 38, 116, 216–18,
219–20; and interpretation of